MICROORGANISM FACTS FOR KIDS

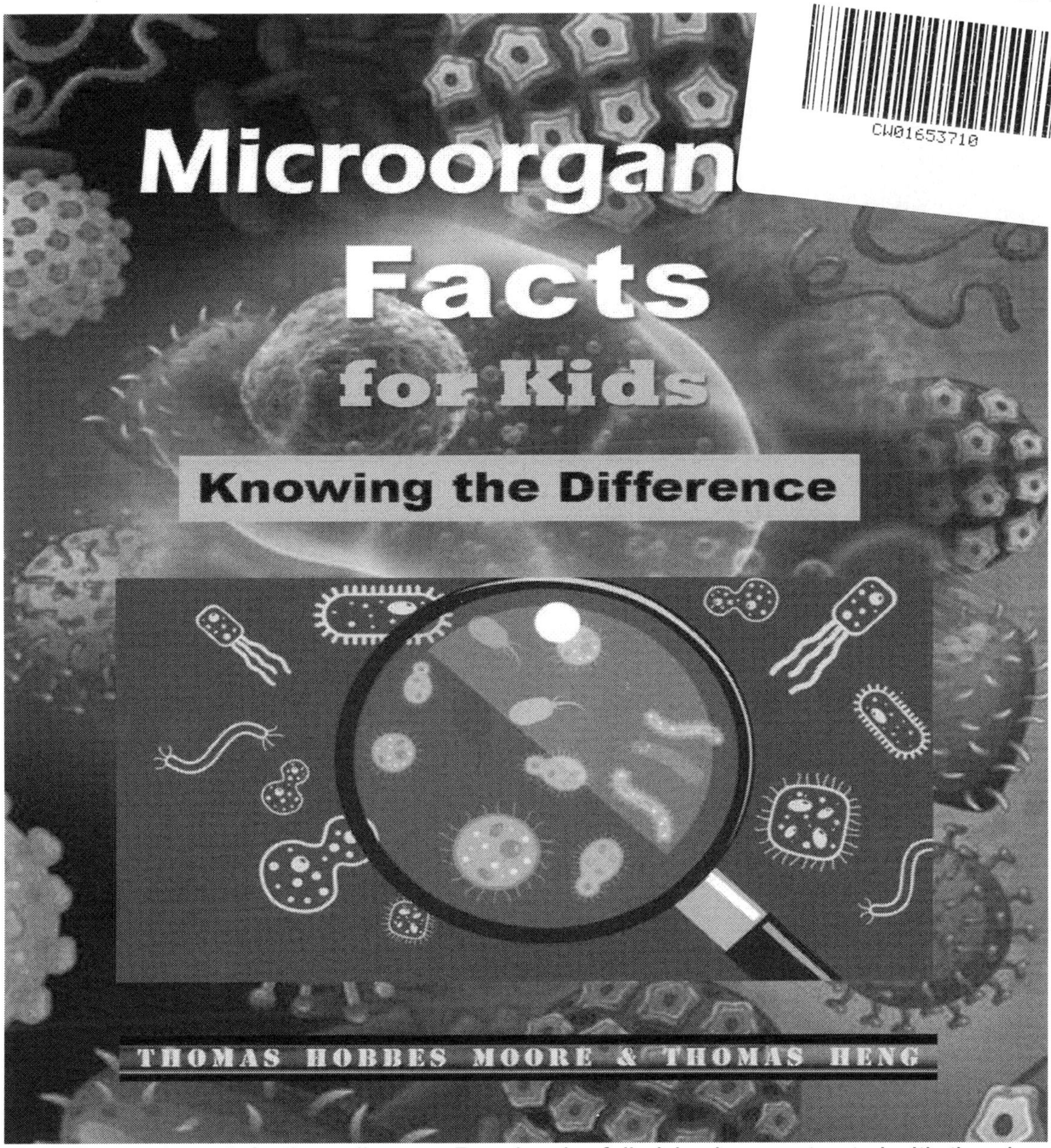

Viral disease is an infectious disease. People who fall sick when contracted with the virus will experience mild to moderate symptoms and then recover from it without any special treatment. This is because the antibodies inside our body fight against the bug if our immune system is healthy and strong. But if it weakened, then the person will succumb to sickness. Antiviral medication is the preferable treatment for viral infection. But to certain illness, it depends on the type of virus that is infecting on that person.

Bacteria are microscopic, single-celled organisms and they come in many shapes and features form ranging from spheres to rods and spirals. They can survive in any diverse environments such as in the soil, the ocean and inside the human gut. Typically, bacteria are considered to be the first life form ever exist on Earth surface, and practically they are around in every habitats' times. There are good and bad bacteria. Good bacteria for instance yogurt can help in our body digestion problems and bad bacteria can cause infections. Human body is more prone to bacterial infections once our body immune system becomes weak. Antibiotics or antibacterial are medications used to treat bacterial infections by killing and reducing the bacteria growth from multiplying inside our body.

Table of Contents

Table of Contents

Microorganism Facts For Kids

Virus Intact On Non-Living Surfaces

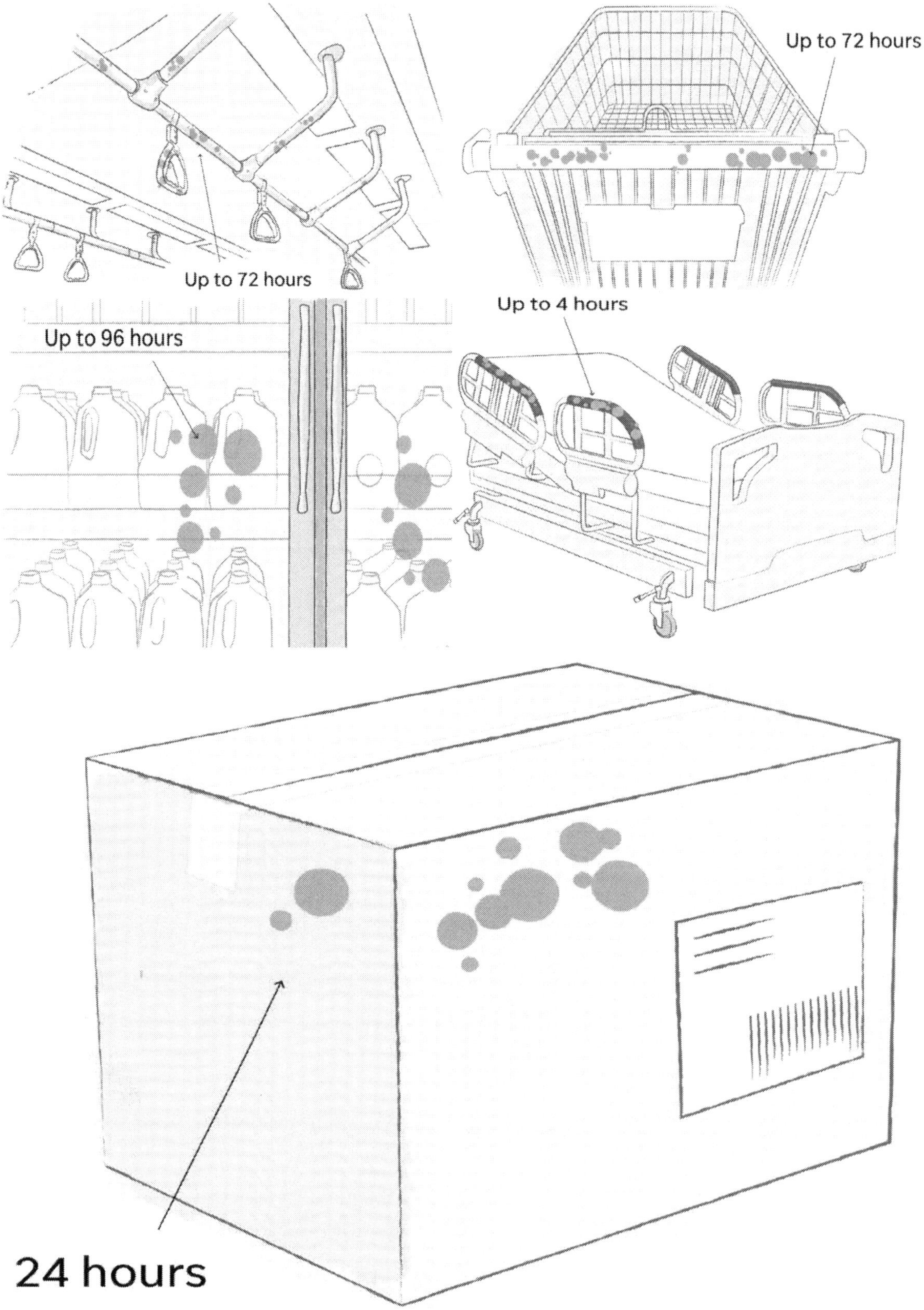

MICROORGANISM FACTS FOR KIDS

Tips to Stay Healthy & Be Safe

Learn the 4 tips to avert potential coronavirus infections from getting into your immune system.

Tip #1 – Practise Good Hygiene

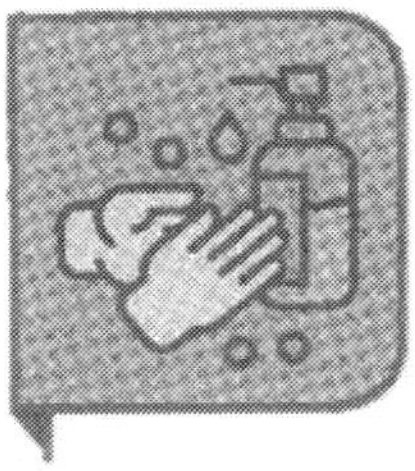

Our hands always come into contact with people, objects and surfaces daily. As most viruses are airborne, washing your hands is equally important. Practise washing your hands for 15 to 30 seconds with soap and water. If water is not within reach, be sure to use hand sanitizers and wipes that brought along with you. They may come in handy at times when you face no water tap or tap malfunctioning at unexpected places.

Tip #2 – Know the Hot Zone and Virus Cluster Areas

Be mindful of "hot zones" or "cluster" areas where infected people come in contact regularly.

Hot zones surface areas for instance handrails, supermarket trolleys and ATMs. Always remember to wash or sanitise your hands after coming into contact with these "hot zones" surface areas. For parents, always remind your children to avoid putting their hands in or near the mouth, nose and face areas when hands always like to touch everywhere and everything on the surface.

Cluster areas where it was made known on local news or social media that infected people had come to visit such places. If need to visit such places, remember to bring along your hand sanitizers and wipes with you. Remind yourself not to use your hands to touch your mouth, nose and face.

Tip #3 – Lead a Healthy Lifestyle

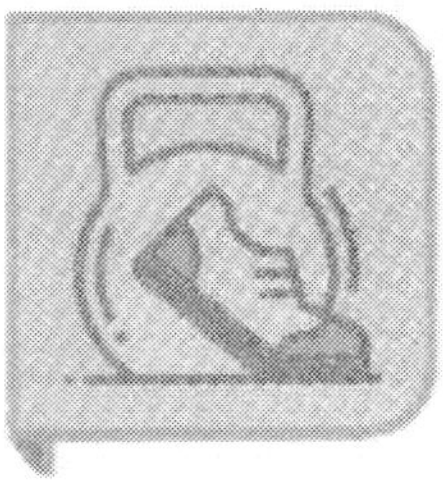

Maintain regular exercise and outdoor activity to keep yourself active and fit and with regular sleep and hydrating yourself by drinking at least sufficient water daily, all these workout hand-in-hand to keep our immunity at optimum levels so that it keeps us strong and fight back against the 'notorious' virus if it comes into attack with our body immune system.

Microorganism Facts For Kids

Tip #4 – Strengthen Yourself with Immunity Boosting Food

Having a balanced diet is essentially important.

Some of the immunity boosting food can derive from our daily food sources are:

1. Ensure each meal intake, there is sufficient amount of vegetables, lean proteins like tofu, fish, chicken etc. and carbohydrates like wholegrain rice.
2. Consider taking varieties of vegetables and fruits to boost our intake of antioxidants.
3. Increasing our intake of Vitamin C. But do not neglect other Vitamin minerals like A, E and D which they are also just as important. Supplements are not necessary if we follow our healthy and balanced diet daily.

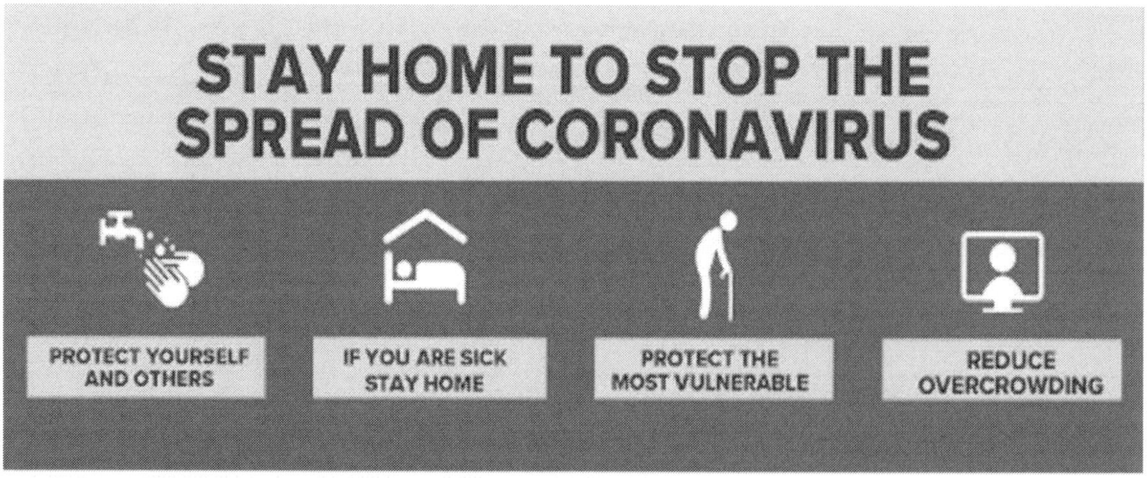
STAY HOME TO STOP THE SPREAD OF CORONAVIRUS
PROTECT YOURSELF AND OTHERS
IF YOU ARE SICK STAY HOME
PROTECT THE MOST VULNERABLE
REDUCE OVERCROWDING

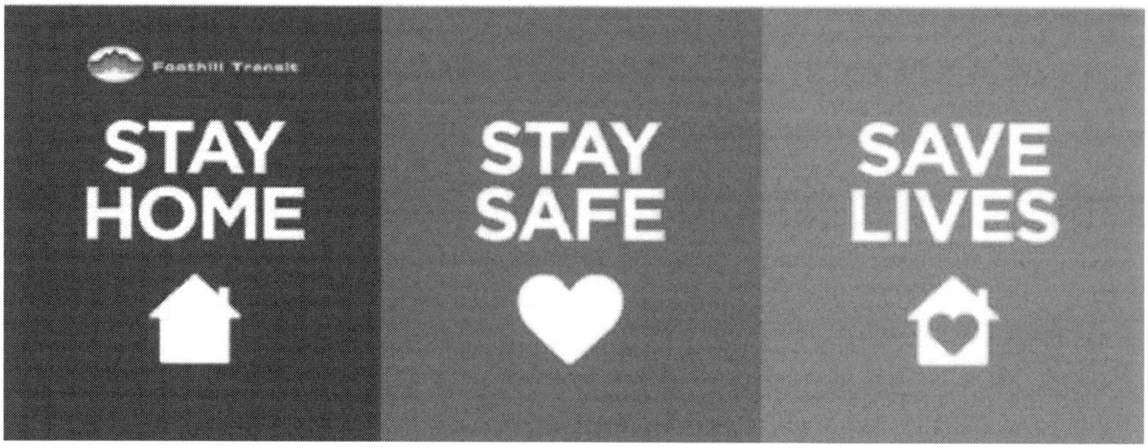
STAY HOME
STAY SAFE
SAVE LIVES

Microorganism Facts For Kids

Helping Children to Cope with COVID-19 Stress

Like adults, kids are also struggling with it. Across the globe, children too will need to follow physical distancing, quarantines if sick and nationwide school closures. Due to the need to stay-at-home measures, there are some who may be feeling more isolated, anxious, and bored, and uncertainty over the school closure as to why there is such fears. From the parents, it triggers down the fear and grief over the impact of the virus onto them. As such, we need to get our children engaged in the understanding of the coronavirus, the challenges it brings to the world and what preventive measures that the country can offer to protect them, us and the citizens.

Keep your children entertain with fun, entertainment and education platforms by watching relevant topics on YouTube and Children TV programmes. Sit beside and teach them to understand the importance of wearing mask, social distancing and safe hand hygiene. Imitate along with the animated characters on TV and learn together with them in particularly the safe hand hygiene by encouraging everyone in the family to participate and wash hands. In this way, it creates fun and excitement for the children to remember some of the important measures need to be followed whenever they are out and about, before and after any meals or snacks.

During lockdown period, introduce readings on social media channels. Encourage them to see books online as a fun, healthy way to make use of their time while at home. But typically limit them to around 30 minutes to an hour maximum and in between break intervals for resting as we do not want to spoil them in spending extended unnecessary hours of viewing on technology gadgets to wilt away their time. Place some other time slots like art and craft for them to have hands-on activities. Or better still, invite them to do some kitchen cooking stuff together with Mum to instil them to think of some brainy dish they like to have for their meal time. All in all, your children will not feel isolated and bored even during school closures as they have mom and dad at home to provide this special moment of time together with them.

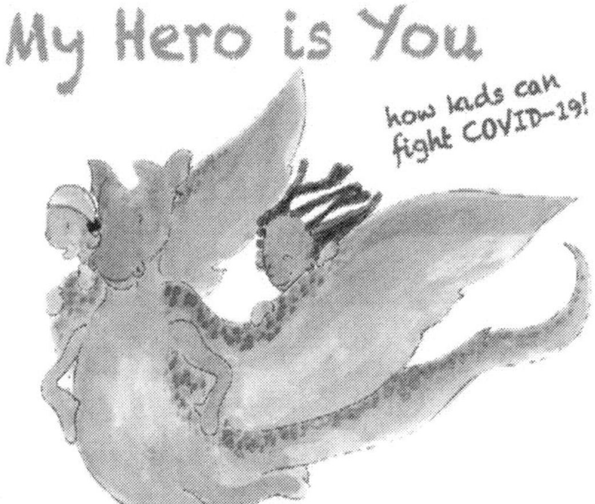

Microorganism Facts For Kids

Fearful of the Global Pandemic Crisis

Everyone is fearful of the deadly virus. Many face stress as isolation, job prospects and family woes get worsen at this time. Schools in many countries are closed. Employees are forced to work from home. Countries go on lockdowns to slow the spread of coronavirus infection.

Many impose strict restrictions and introduce three phases in the lockdowns to gradually ease and lift up each phase where people can resume back to work, but for some companies the remote work still remain norm for their office staffs. They are asked to continue the use of interconnecting and virtual communications over Zoom video connectivity platform as part of the business operations continuity to interact with internal managements, customers and suppliers.

When city starts to intensify more movement restrictions in line with the increasing number of coronavirus infection cases, many companies may file more bankruptcy and more people will lose their jobs and ultimately in the end many will suffer anxieties and depression over financial difficulties in supporting a family.

But in every crisis, there lies opportunities in others.

People can cancel holiday plans, travel less and stop social gatherings but normal life will still have to go on as usual. Even if everyone in the family have to stay at home, we still need to cook and eat, children will still need to study and people still need to exercise to keep fit and stay healthy. Basic essentials like food, clothes, and household items like toilet paper are some of the needs that people will need to have them while on lockdowns.

The situation is rapidly changing. As more cities are going under lockdowns, non-essential businesses are ordered to close and consumers are generally avoiding crowded places for fear of getting infected.

More and more people are now turning to shop online instead of in stores as it can be seen that E-commerce stores are getting a spike of 300% more online sales in just over a week based on statistical data.

Many industries are falling because of the virus - Airline, Tourism, Hotels and Sport. But yet E-commerce sector alongside with goods delivery businesses are booming like crazy and will grow further even after the virus is gone.

Microorganism Facts For Kids

Generally speaking, a new business trend is already taking shape and will change the whole world of how we do and negotiate businesses in a new era dimension.

Traditional business model will have to be remodel and re-strategized to fit in in order to sustain its business continuation while keeping their workplace safe and establishing new ways to get employees to work from home to become a permanent part of their business operations.

Nobody knows when will this crisis be ending but even before everything goes back to normalcy, we better get ourselves brace up and prepare for the upcoming recession affected by the virus. There will be no quick return to how things were as before. The virus is resilient and hard to eradicate it without effective vaccine.

Lives and the ways of approaching it to combat this coronavirus transmission must continue to adapt and evolve along with the pandemic as it goes until one day an effective vaccine is developed to treat it.

Meanwhile, this entails our new way of living for the foreseeable future with an extended new norm of social distancing and mask wearing applicable in our daily lifestyle even as lockdowns are eased and restriction measures are gradually lifted up in phases.

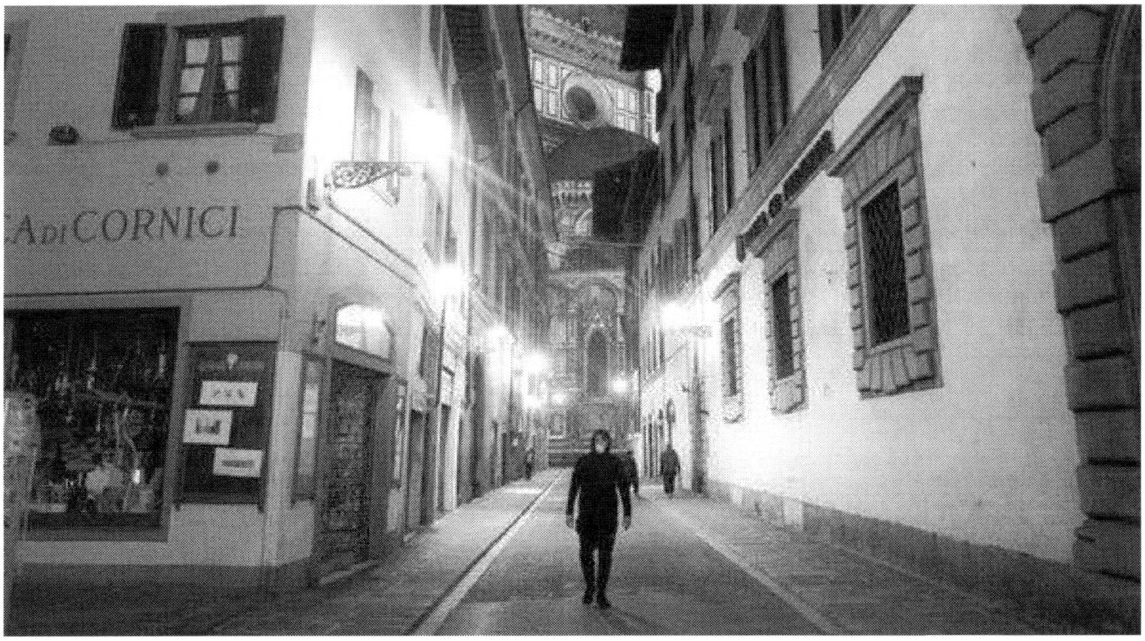

Already, countries like Japan, China and South Korea had seen struggling with imported infection cases after they eased their lockdowns to restart their economies and resuming their airline travel sectors.

MICROORGANISM FACTS FOR KIDS

Many people are still susceptible to the virus transmission as long as they have not been infected by the virus, they are still not immune to it yet. If they did not take the social distancing measures seriously, they will be vulnerable to the virus transmission and get infected as well.

Notwithstanding all the inconveniences created by the pandemic impacts, immunisation programmes against other diseases like polio, measles and rubella must not be disrupted for those who are in need.

All in all, the medical experts bluntly put it to the fact that coronavirus transmission will continue to occur for some time even if one country succeeds in containing it, it will still give rise to new outbreaks as it keeps arriving from somewhere else!

We must brace ourselves up for the next waves of coronavirus infections as many had still not learned enough from the past mistakes of not taking it seriously on the social distancing and mask wearing preventive measures. Until the day we had truly learned the importance of these adoption of tough measures being implemented, there will continue to be new infections and countless of innocent deaths occurred due to the stubbornness behavioural patterns of some other people.

In the meantime, take good care of yourself and adopt these measures to protect yourself and others as well. Wash your hands frequently with soap, use and bin tissues when coughing or sneezing. Avoid touching your eyes, nose and mouth when out and about. Stay safe and be stress free!

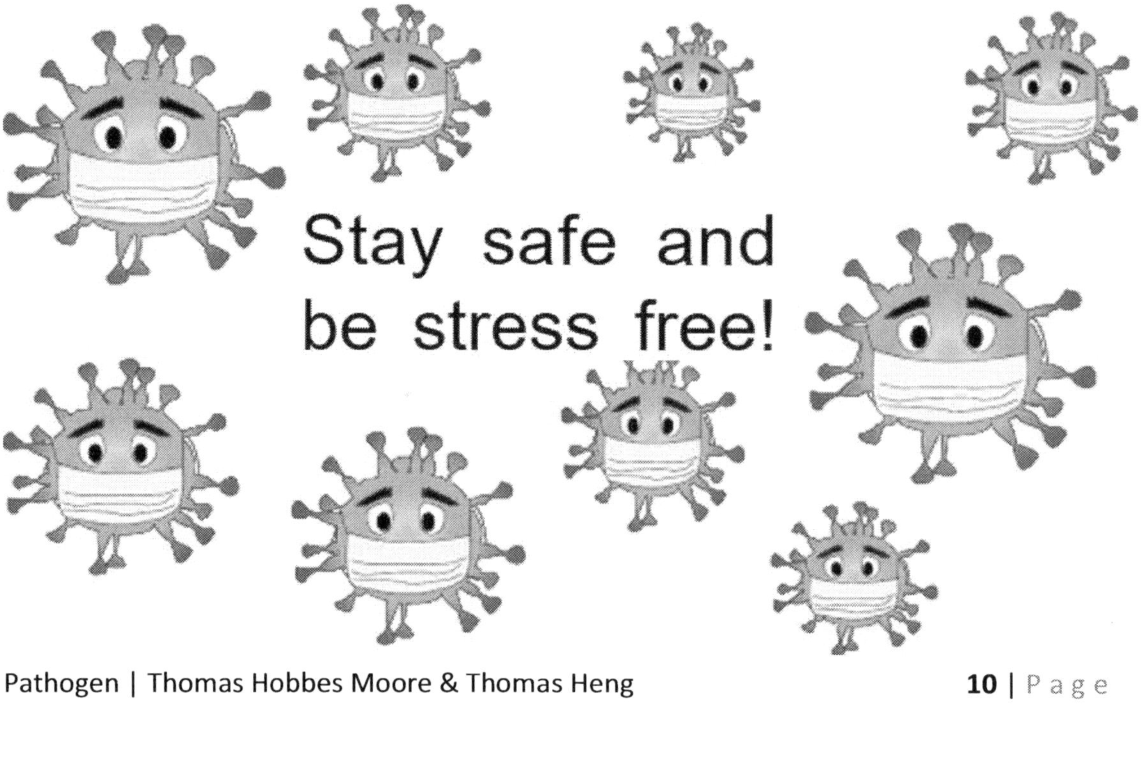

Microorganism Facts For Kids

Microorganism Facts for Kids

Microorganism is also known as microbe which cannot be seen by our naked eye. It can only be seen under a microscope. It belongs to a diverse group of minute and simple form of living cells which include bacteria, algae, fungi, protozoa and viruses. They live almost everywhere and around us. They are in our soil, the drinking water, the air we breathe in, on our skin, in our bodies etc. where they get their source of energy in many different ways.

They may be either free-living microorganisms that help to break it down into natural chemicals which are useful in our environment or parasites that live by invading good living cells and cause disease to spread and invade our central nervous system to make us fall severely ill.

Bacteria are single-celled microorganisms. They don't have nucleus but have cell walls similar to plant cells and come in many shape forms which include rods, spirals and spheres. Some bacteria behavioural patterns look just like long tail "swimming" around while others just like to glide along.

Viruses always reproduce inside other living things. They cannot simply live on its own. They need to invade the host cell, replicate it and then multiply it to further invading on other host cells again to repeat its cycle.

Other types of microbes are useful to nutrients recycle in ecosystems by acting as decomposers. For example fallen leaves and dead animals whereby they feed and cause them to breakdown or decay to mix with our soil to provide essential nutrients to the needs of our living plants. Without this natural process, the nutrients in the soil will run out and our plants will not be able to stay and looks healthy. Hence, they are also our natural recyclers of living things on Earth.

All animals have bacteria and protozoa living on them without doing any harm. So are humans too when inside our human gut, there lies even more bacterial cells than other living human cells. These organisms are vital to help us in our food digestion when food had consumed and travelled into our gut system to perform its functions. There are around 500 to 1000 different types of bacteria inhabit our mouth. Most people think that microbes are dangerous but in fact they are not. Some even benefit our body to produce antibodies inside our immune system to fight against bad pathogens.

MICROORGANISM FACTS FOR KIDS

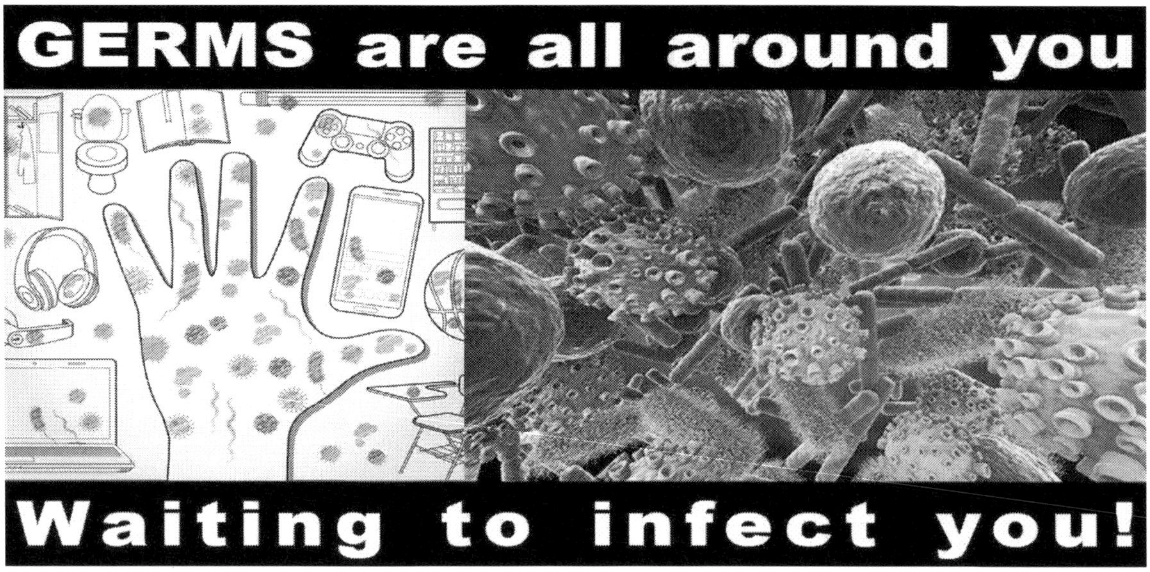

Any unhygienic person can just pick up the germs. The germ virus penetrates its way into the body immune system to reach the host cell. It then starts to "hack" the cell relentlessly and replicate copies of itself to release even more viruses to make its way to attack and destroy all other good cells through the body, making the person fall seriously ill as a result.

Pay close attention to our elderly who are most vulnerable to the virus attack, particularly in their personal hygiene at this time of crisis. We must ensure they drink sufficient water daily, stay indoors and help them monitor their temperature twice daily to keep them safe from the virus. Attend to their needs, chit-chatting and keeping them happy can address their anxieties that are likely to emerge as they spend a lot of time alone at home as a result of cancelled social activities and boredom at home.

Generally an increase in stress is actually a normal response. However it is also be unpleasant in another form that can hinder their immunity to fight against the deadly virus.

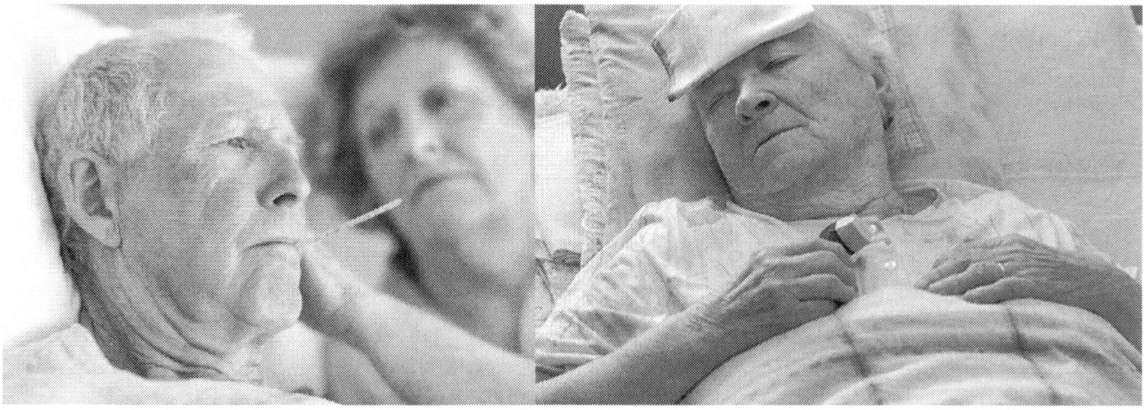

Microorganism Facts For Kids

Booster Required Even COVID-19 Vaccine Is Ready

Human trials have begun its course to get it tested on humans and to get ready with the cure and reverse the pandemic back to normalcy and to reshape the economy health.

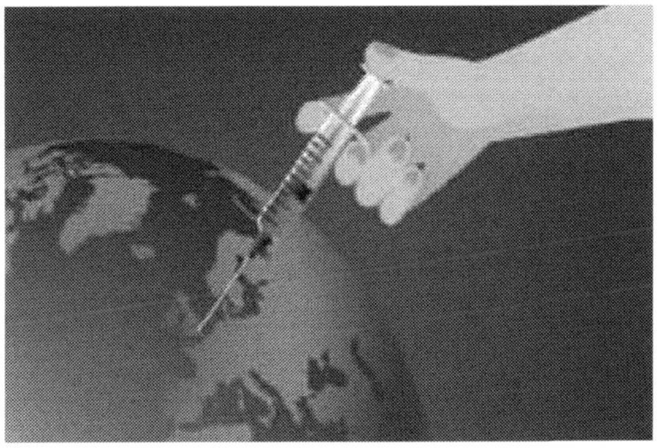

But nevertheless experts warn that even if the human trials go well and a vaccine cure is found, there are still many barriers basically evolving around countries and billions of people before global immunisations become feasible for every one of us to be safe from the coronavirus episode.

In general, most viruses in the past seem to have long-lasting memories in a person's immune system but encountering this new virus, COVID-19, this will not be the same case anymore.

Infectious experts, scientists and doctors alike share the same sentiments from the studies based on these symptom onsets. It is more likely that even if the most potential vaccines have been created to protect and prevent the coronavirus infection, it will still require boosters and perhaps regularly!

Why is it so?

When an infectious pathogen sneaks into our body by chance, human immune system will automatically recognise the germ patterns and create a memory. The next time when the immune system comes across the same germ patterns again, it will automatically make a quick and repelling response to fight against it. If it wins, the person will not fall ill or just getting a mild symptom instead.

In most infectious viruses' case, natural infection is the best preventive alternatives to give a long-lasting memory to a human immune system if possibly to have it to totally eradicate out the infectious pathogens. But in COVID-19, it is not always the case.

Therefore, the whole idea of making the vaccine to become effective inside the human body is to give the victim a version of the infectious pathogen that will not have cause the disease and make the person sick but instead creating an immune system memory to it. This theory is similar to the vaccines that were developed for measles, mumps and rubella (MMR). It contains live but disabled versions of the dead virus inside the human body.

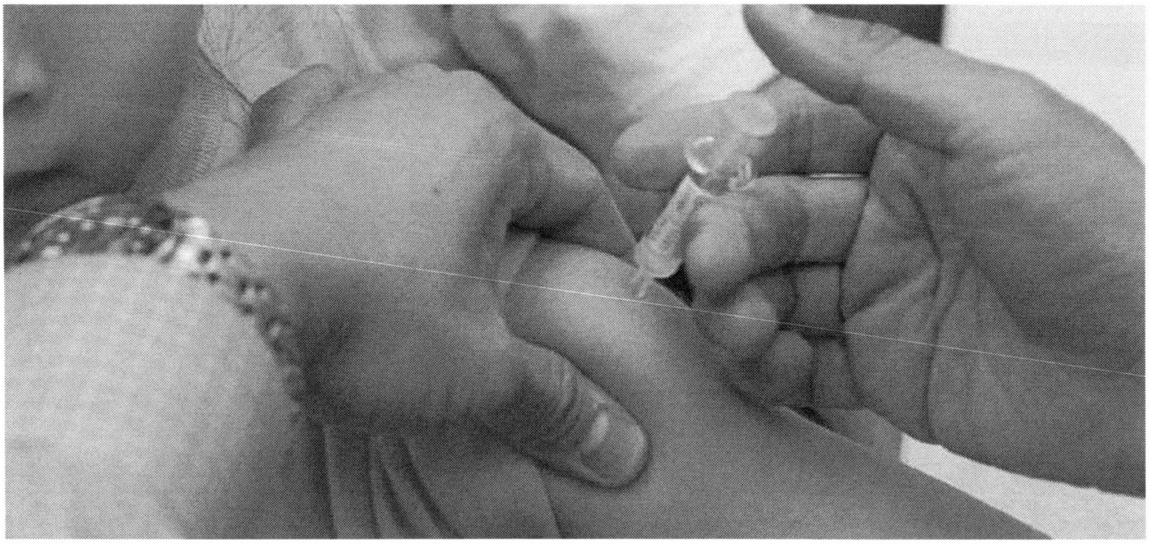

Children are generally given two doses of the vaccine a few years apart. So, in this case if the vaccine does not remember the first time round, their immune system can still remind how the virus look like in the second round of the immunisation vaccination. Nevertheless, pre-school child's immune system is generally still developing until they have reached the age of 7.

Normally, it takes years before a safe and effective live vaccine can be developed and distributed for healthcare medical professionals to endorse in their immunisation vaccination process. Researchers are now trying different means and route of approach to the killer disease. A good approach is whereby making use of a killed version of the virus rather than a modified and live version of a virus as in the case of MMR.

For examples both the polio and influenza vaccines make use of killed viruses. The main drawback of using killed viruses as vaccine is that the immune response does not stay lasting inside our human body and that is why booster will have to come in to repeat the course again. Each year, boosters need to be injected to keep stimulating the immune memory because the infectious virus in the vaccine is not live. They need to be reminded of how they the virus patterns look like. In an event of an outbreak situation occurs again, the local community will have every person in close contact within the affected area to go for a dose of the vaccine in order to contain the transmission and reduce the spread of the virus to elsewhere.

MICROORGANISM FACTS FOR KIDS

Learning More about Pathogen

A pathogen is a bacterium, virus, germ, or other micro-organism that can cause infectious diseases.

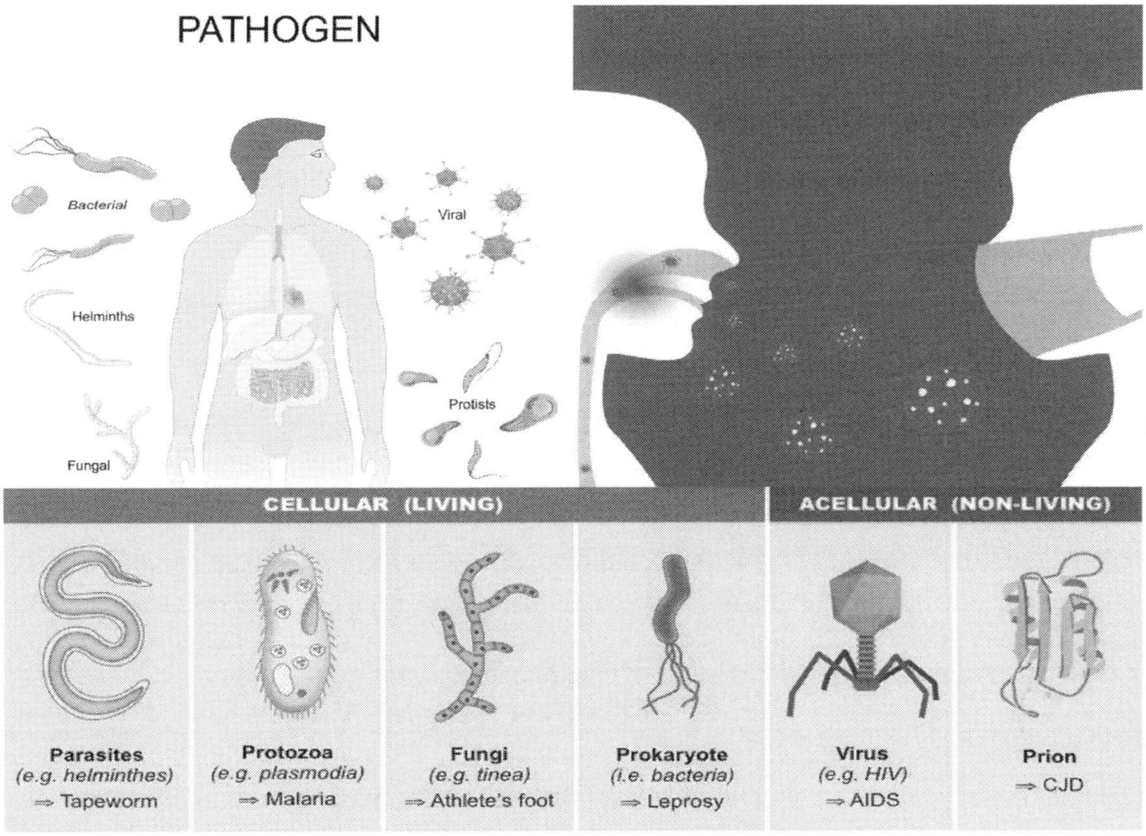

Typically, germs inside our body cannot cause any harmful effects because of our healthy body immunity system that automatically respond and fighting against the bacteria that comes along its way.

However, if we were to suffer an illness, then our immune system will be weakened. These microbes will be then have a greater chance to sneak into our body organs through the passageway of our nostrils via our hands touching the eyes, putting inside our mouth or open wound that breaches through our skin layer's barriers.

Some diseases can be spread through direct contact with another person who had infected skin, mucous membranes, or by their bodily fluids like coughing and sneezing out and by sexually transmitted diseases like AIDS. A human pathogen can make a person feel very ill and devastating, and sometimes even fatal and life threatening.

The main types of pathogens are:

MICROORGANISM FACTS FOR KIDS

1. Viruses

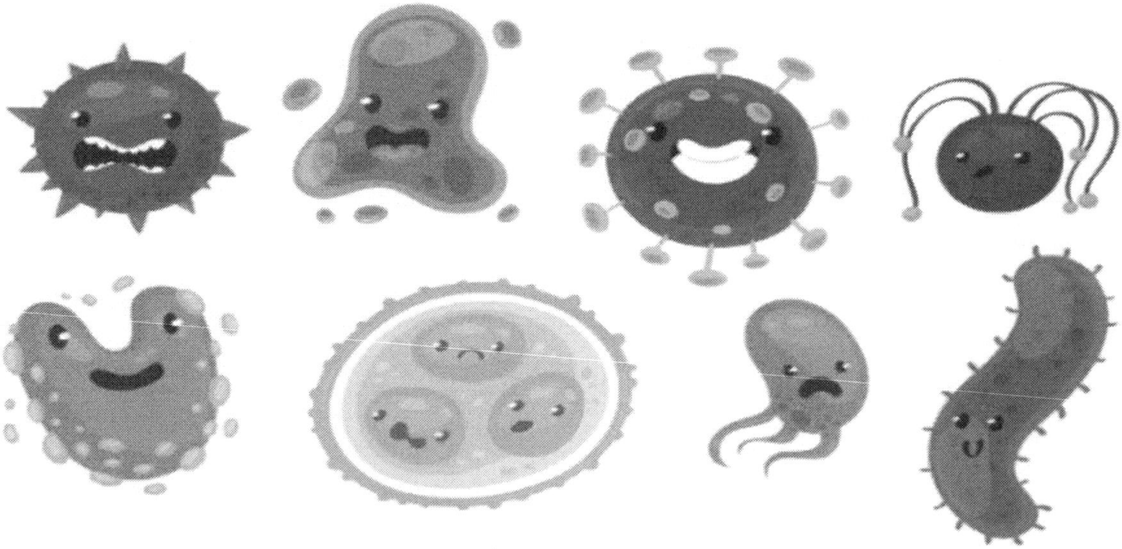

Viruses are microscopic parasites or refer to microorganisms which are much tinnier than bacteria in form. They can make humans sick but they cannot do anything on their own unlike bacteria. They simply need to live inside another creature that is on their neighbouring host cell in order to survive.

To do that, they have to get out and infect into our human cells. The virus particle can stays intact and thrive on the surface for a period of approximately 12 hours up to several days while waiting to infect another person of suitable organism that comes in contact with the surface. Once the person touches the contaminated surface area, he will pick up the virus. In seconds, the virus spreads into his whole body and soon it turns to a reservoir of virus particles to grow and multiply freely at a rapid speed.

While coughing and sneezing, droplets of it will go into airborne transmission. Either it is inhaled by another person who just happened to be nearby the area or it can even land on any other non-living surface and waiting for another person to accidentally touch on it and gets infected.

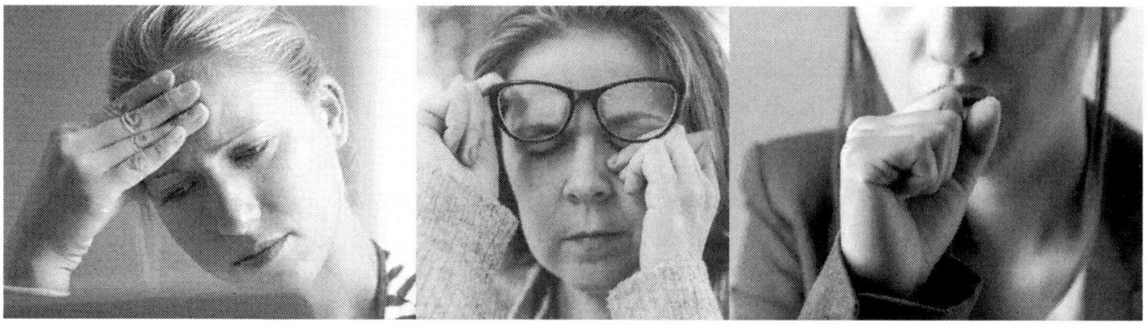

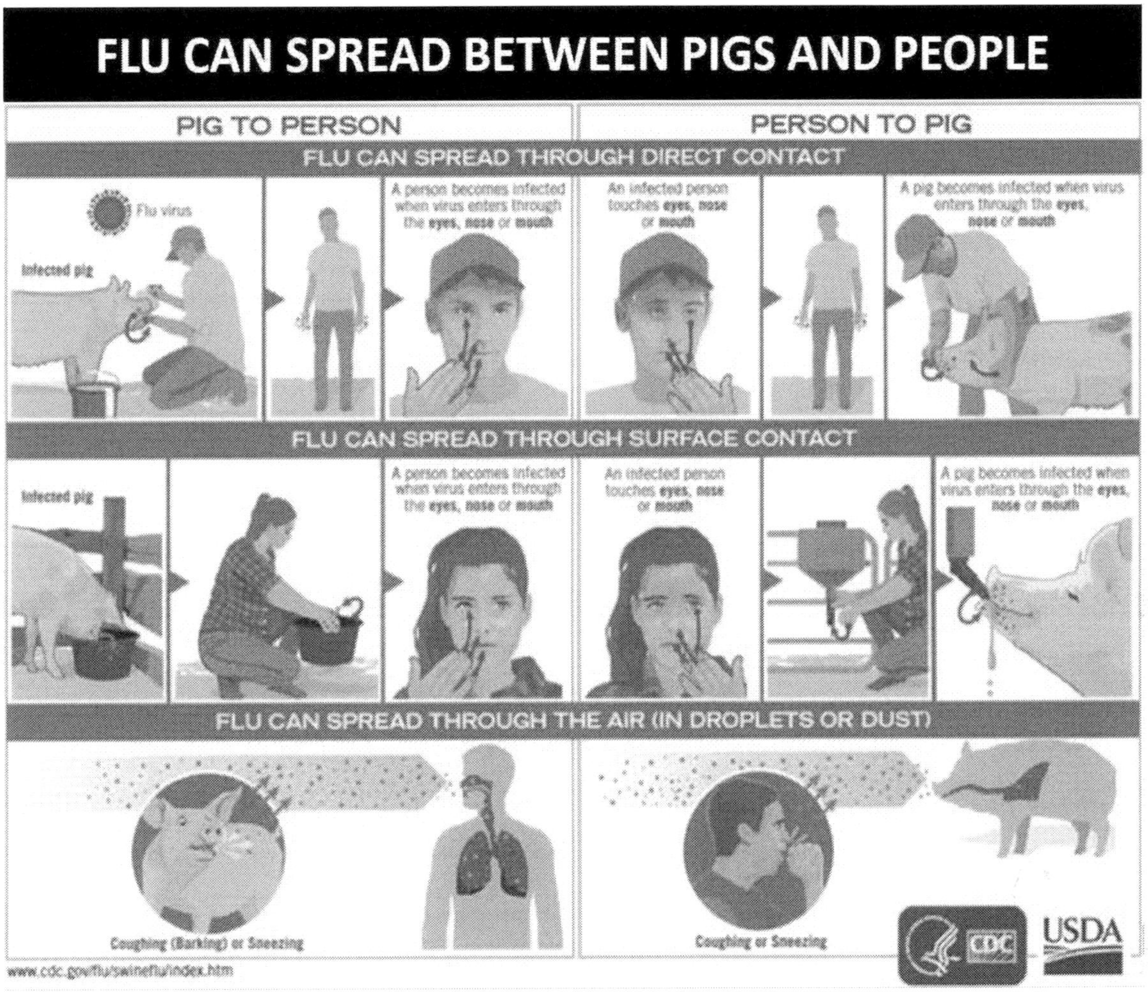

There are some reported cases stating that those recovered from the viral infection can still fall sick again. The reason given by the medical expert is that not all viruses are totally eradicated from the person body yet when they initially recovered. Some are still left behind but stay dormant inside their body for a short period of time without causing any negative effects before they restart and multiply itself again.

Medical experts was shocked to discover that this new virus, COVID-19, can also perform mutations in many combination and can even combine with another infected cell as well.

Impending COVID-19 Vaccine

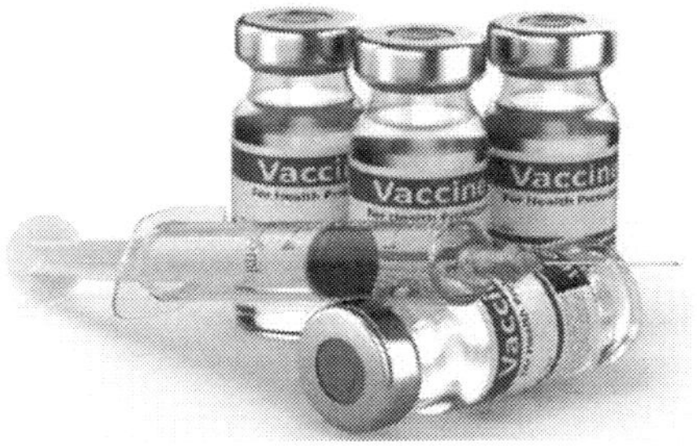

Furthermore, this virus affects differently on different ethnic group and it makes the vaccine task even more difficult to develop to have a single effective dose treatment cure for all.

Microorganism Facts For Kids

Viral Diseases

A viral disease or **viral infection** occurs when microorganisms enter a human body and causes infections by continuing to invade the immune system until its susceptible cells break down and cause the person to fall severely ill.

Influenza is a viral infection. It occurs at the upper respiratory tract area from nose, throat and lungs pathways. For example a common cold illness. For most people, influenza can resolve and recover on its own. Influenza is not the same as stomach flu viruses where it can make the person to have consistent diarrhoea and vomiting throughout the episodes.

Overview of Viral Infections

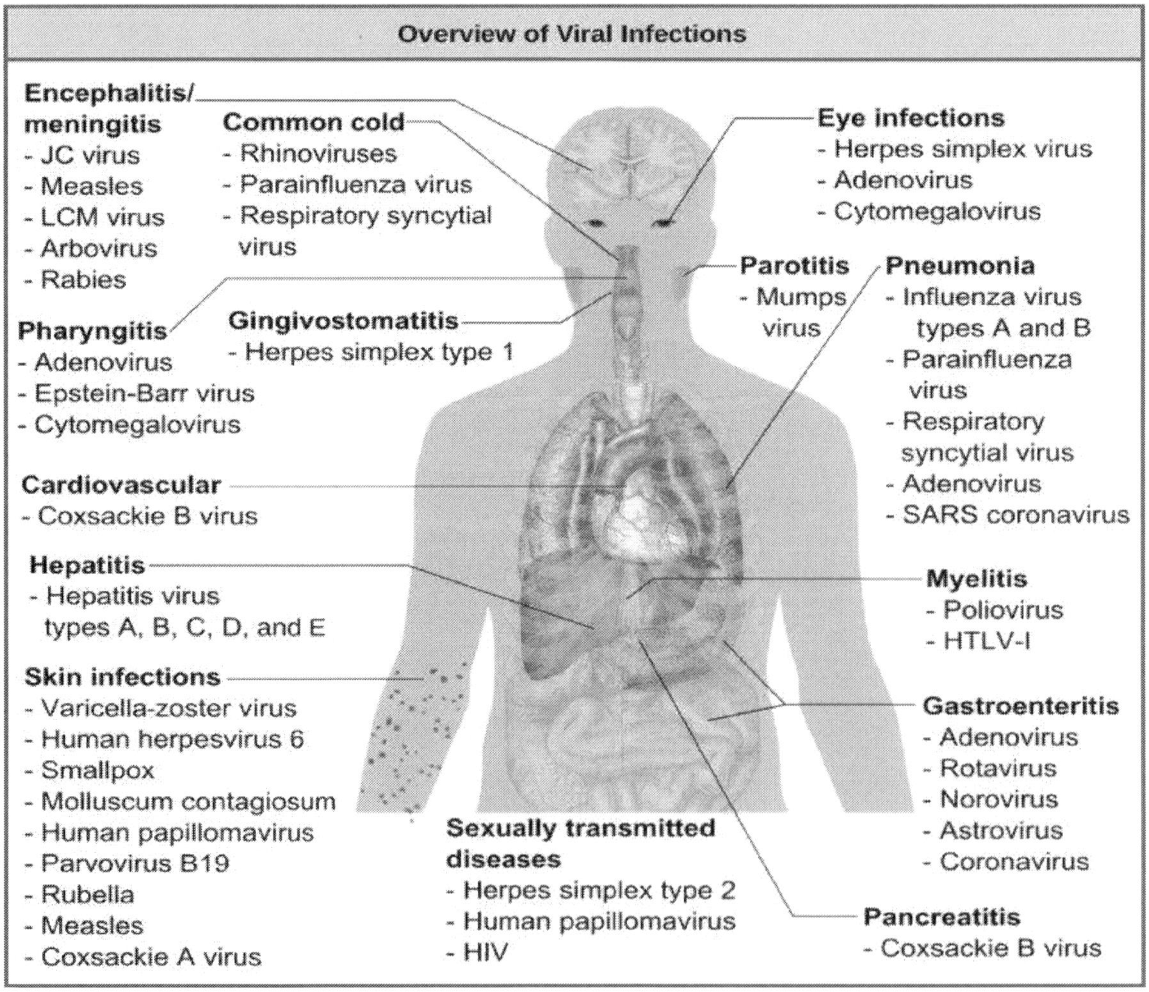

Generally, antibiotics are used to treat bacteria symptoms but not viruses. Antibiotic medications does not work against viral infections. Antiviral medication is the only effective medication work for treating viral infections.

MICROORGANISM FACTS FOR KIDS

Influenza is commonly known as "flu". It is an infectious disease caused by an influenza virus and their symptoms range from mild to severe. It can make the person to run high fever, runny nose, sore throat, muscle and joint pain, headache, coughing and feeling tired. Neuraminidase drugs are to treat this type of antiviral infection and work effectively well if it is taken within a day or two once the onset symptom appears.

Examples of viral diseases include:

- Common cold
- Flu
- Meningitis
- Warts, including genital warts
- Oral and Genital herpes
- Chickenpox/Shingles
- Measles
- Viral Gastroenteritis, including Norovirus and Rotavirus
- Hepatitis A, B, C, D, E
- Yellow Fever
- Dengue Fever
- HIV and AIDS

Symptoms of Viral Infections

Some symptoms include:

FEVER	MUSCLE ACHES	COUGHING	SNEEZING
RUNNY NOSE	HEADACHE	CHILLS	DIARRHEA

Condition	Cause	Use an Antibiotic?
Strep throat	Bacteria	**Yes.** Your provider will prescribe one for your infection.
Whooping cough	Bacteria	
Urinary tract infection	Bacteria	
★ Sinus infection	Bacteria or Virus	**Maybe.** Your provider can tell if an antibiotic will help.
Middle ear infection	Bacteria or Virus	
Bronchitis/chest cold *(in an otherwise healthy person)*	Bacteria or Virus	**No.** Bronchitis is rarely caused by bacteria.
Common cold	Virus	**No.** Viral infections don't respond to antibiotics. Ask your provider how to treat your symptoms.
Sore throat	Virus	
Flu	Virus	
Asthma	Virus	

Thera are four types of influenza viruses, namely A, B, C and D type. Influenza A and B viruses commonly affect humans when come near in contact with infected swine (pigs) carrying the disease. Influenza C infections primarily cause mild upper respiratory tract illness and is extremely rare in human cases that occurred in lower respiratory tract complications. To-date, there is no vaccine that can treat influenza C virus. Influenza D viruses primarily infect pigs and cattle. So far in medical history, no human infection cases had ever recorded from this virus.

MICROORGANISM FACTS FOR KIDS

Seasonal flu vaccines do not protect against influenza C and D viruses' infection and is considered a one type of influenza vaccine make to treat all influenza-like symptoms as there are other viruses too that can result in influenza-like illness spread during the flu season. The most common antiviral medications are Oseltamivir (under the brand name of Tamiflu) and Zanamivir (Relenza).

A. Oseltamivir drugs (Tamiflu)

This type of drugs usually shorten the recovery time for those suffer from flu symptoms such as stuffy or runny nose, sore throat, cough, muscle or joint aches, tiredness, headache, fever, and chills. It is commonly used to treat influenza A and B.

Tamiflu Oseltamivir Medication

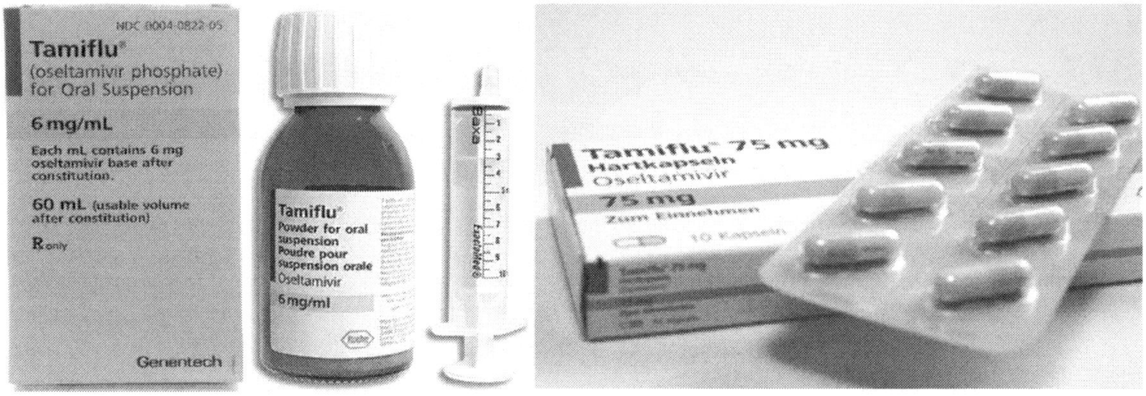

B. Zanamivir (Relenza)

It is a neuraminidase inhibitor. Its treatment is to prevent infections from influenza A (H1N1) and is an effective inhaler to treat flu symptoms victims. Usually after using it, they are likely to feel better after one or two days.

Zanamivir Oral Inhalation Medication

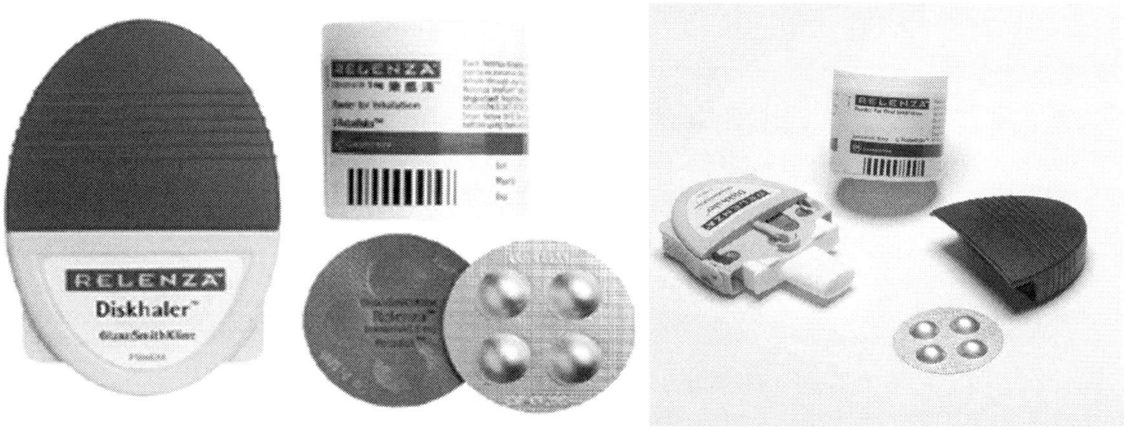

MICROORGANISM FACTS FOR KIDS

2. Bacterial Infections

Bacteria are single-celled microbes. They come in many shapes and forms. Its features range from spheres to rods and spirals.

The internal cell structure has no nucleus, but only the DNA core is surrounded by two protective covering layers which is the outer cell wall and an inner cell membrane.

Mycoplasmas bacterial does not have any cell wall enclosure, but they can inhibit additional third outermost protective layer instead of two covering layers.

Bacteria reside in human intestinal gut and can also live in any adverse environment such as in the soil and water too.

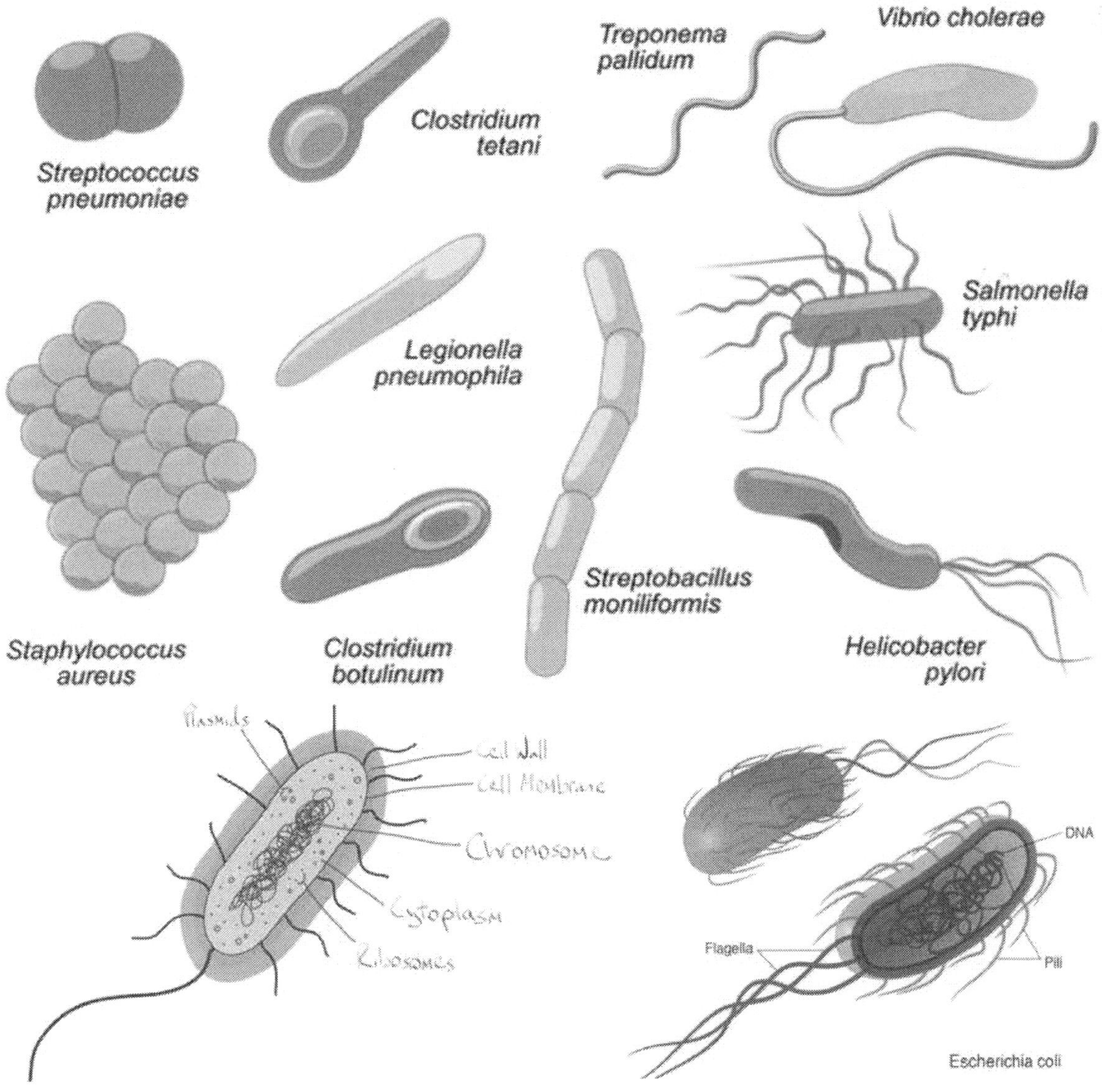

MICROORGANISM FACTS FOR KIDS

Bacteria are considered to be the first life form ever exist on the Earth surface.

There are good and bad bacteria.

Good bacteria for example yogurt is good for treating digestion related problems.

Bad bacteria cause infections.

Our human body is prone to bacterial infections if the immune function is weakened.

Antibiotics or antibacterial are medications used to treat bacterial infections by killing and reducing the bacteria growth from multiplying inside our body.

They come in many physical packaging form such as in tablets, pill capsules, liquids, creams and ointments for wounds.

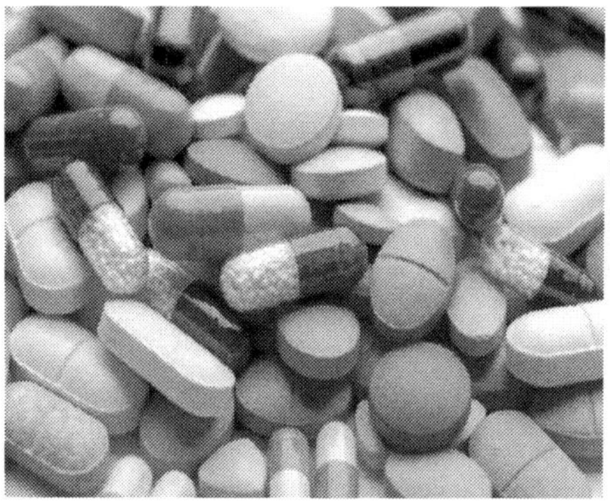

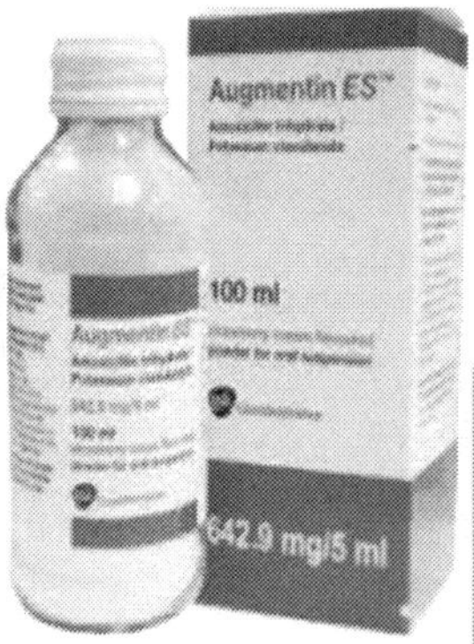

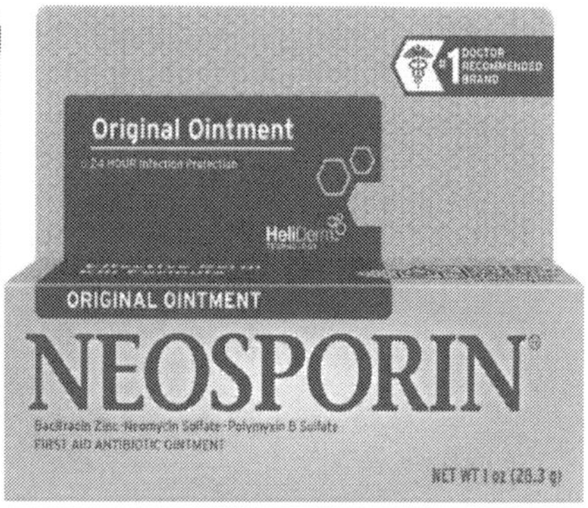

Antibiotics can only be prescribed by doctor.

They must not overconsume and need to adhere strictly according to his prescription.

Overconsuming can cause reverse resistant effect to the bacterial treatment in our body to develop an immunity to fight against the same kind of bacterial symptoms.

When future illness comes with the same bacterial symptoms, the medication can no longer work effectively anymore because the antibiotic resistance had been build up inside our immune system to react upon it.

That explains why doctors don't always prescribe antibiotics treatment for patients unless necessary or his illness doesn't show any improvement after taking the standard flu medication.

How antibiotic resistance develops

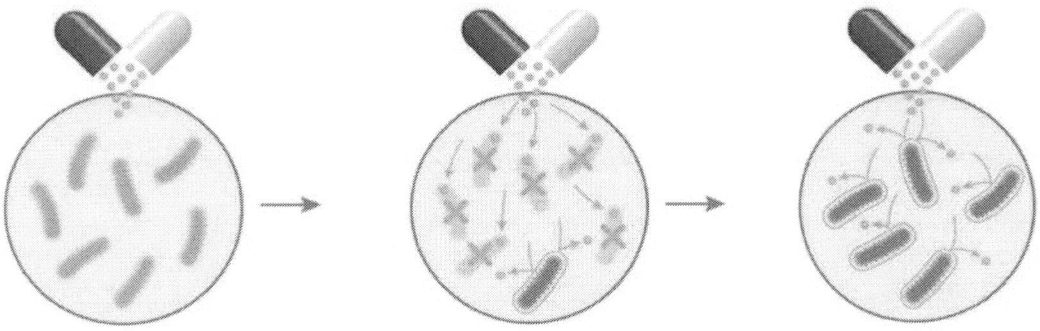

Antibiotics help our bodies To kill the types of bacteria that make us sick

Some of the bacteria that makes us sick get better at defending themselves against antibiotics, meaning resistant bacteria are harder to kill. This is called antibiotic resistance

The resistant bacteria start to multiply, making our antibiotics less and less effective

Some of the bacterial infections are:

- Bacterial Gastroenteritis (salmonella food poisoning or E.coli infection)
- Lyme disease (Insect bites)
- Urinary tract infection (UTI)
- Strep throat
- Bacterial Meningitis
- Gonorrhoea (HIV)
- Cellulitis
- TB, Tuberculosis

Bacterial Infections

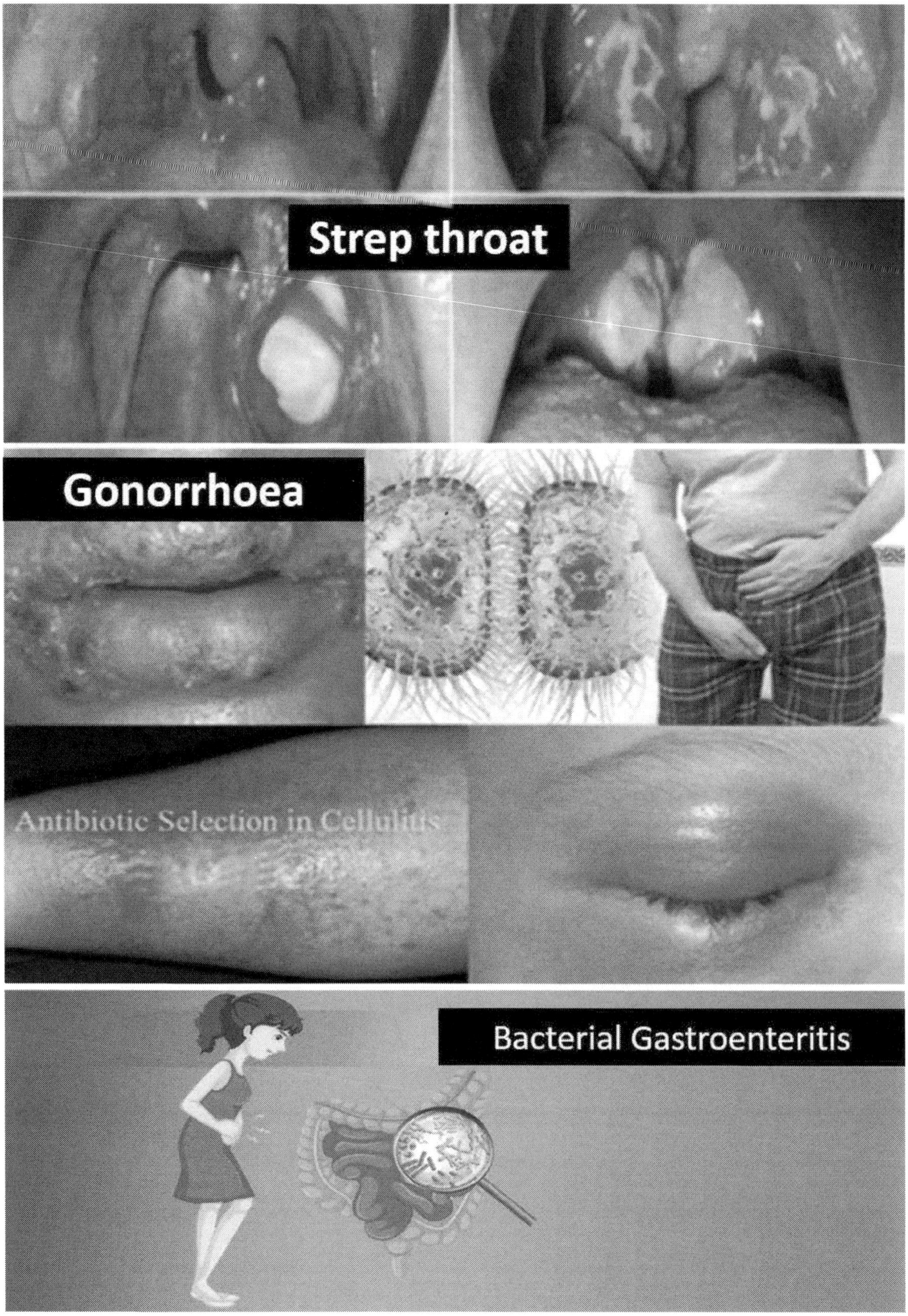

MICROORGANISM FACTS FOR KIDS

Bacteria versus Virus

Bacteria

- Bacteria are larger than viruses.
- They are capable to reproduce and multiply on its own.

Virus

- Viruses are much smaller than bacteria
- They cannot reproduce on their own.
- Their reproduction is by infecting a host cell and making use of the host's DNA repair and replication systems to make copies of itself.

After replication had completed, they leave the host cell and start to infect the neighbouring host cell and the reproduction cycle repeats again.

Influenza symptoms can be mild to severe.

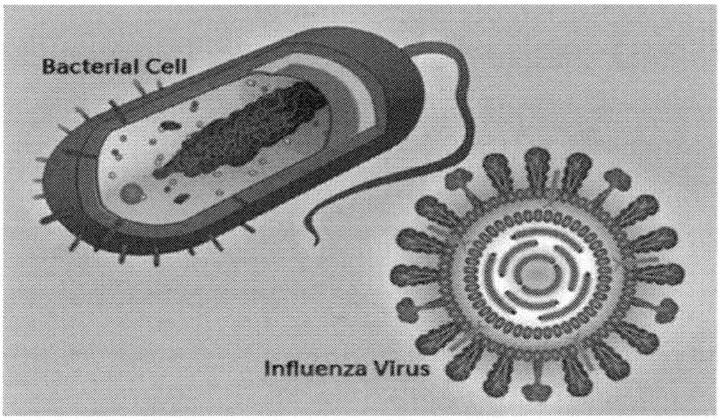

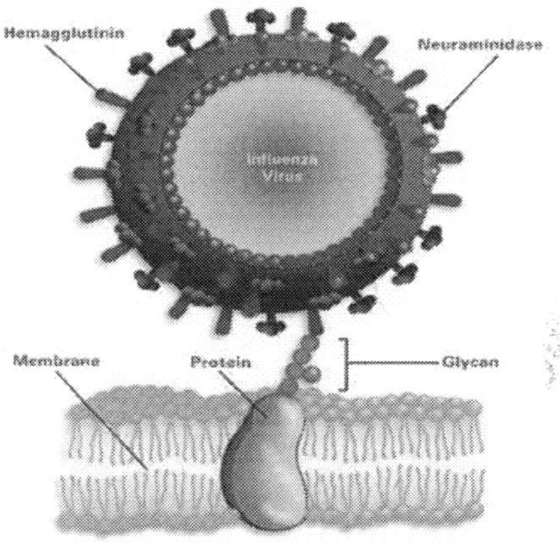

Viruses have no nucleus, cytoplasm, organelles, or cell membrane, so can not carry out cellular functions. Only able to replicate by infecting cells and using the organelles and enzymes
very small, size
Consists of two parts: a nucleic acid and a protein coat called a capsid
Nucleic acid may be DNA or RNA but not both.

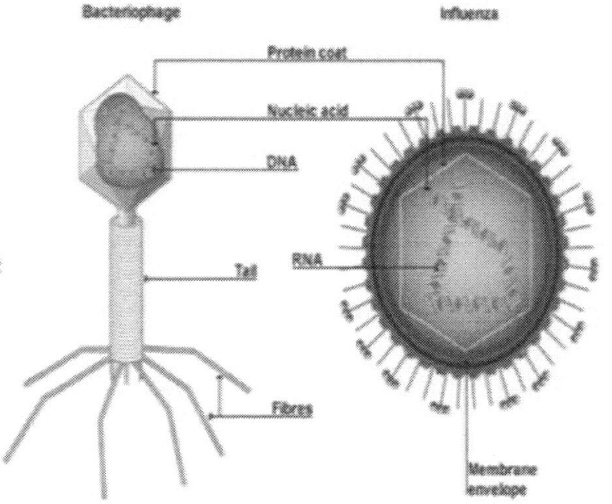

3. Fungal infections

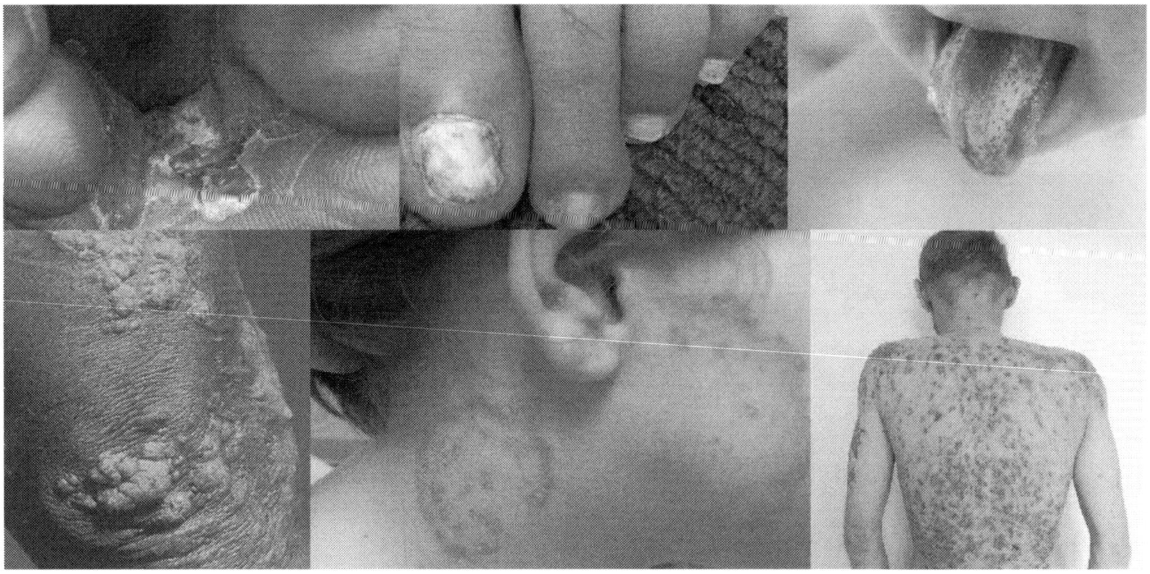

They come from contaminated food and water.

By improper cleaning habits after handling contaminated food, these germs such as E. coli and Salmonella can sneak through and penetrate into our body's digestive system.

Fungi cells usually consist of a nucleus with a protective membrane and a thick cell wall, and thus making it harder to kill. They can colonise and live on and inside our body to multiply many times out of control and cause an infection when they overgrow and appear visibly on our skin in many parts of our body.

For example athlete's foot, woman with a vaginal yeast infection etc.

Basically, they can affect any living and non-living things and everywhere in our environment. For example non-living surfaces such as indoors and outdoors besides infecting on human skin tissues.

Those who are having athlete's foot causes itchiness, scaly rashes on the feet or in between their toes especially sweaty feet people who often wear closed-toed, occlusive shoes.

Some examples of fungal infections are Jock itch, Ringworm, Yeast infection and Onychomycosis (refers to nail fungal infection).

There are exceptional cases where fungal infection does not only cause infections in humans, they can also cause severe illness for those who are diabetic and had weaker body immune systems.

4. Parasitic Infections

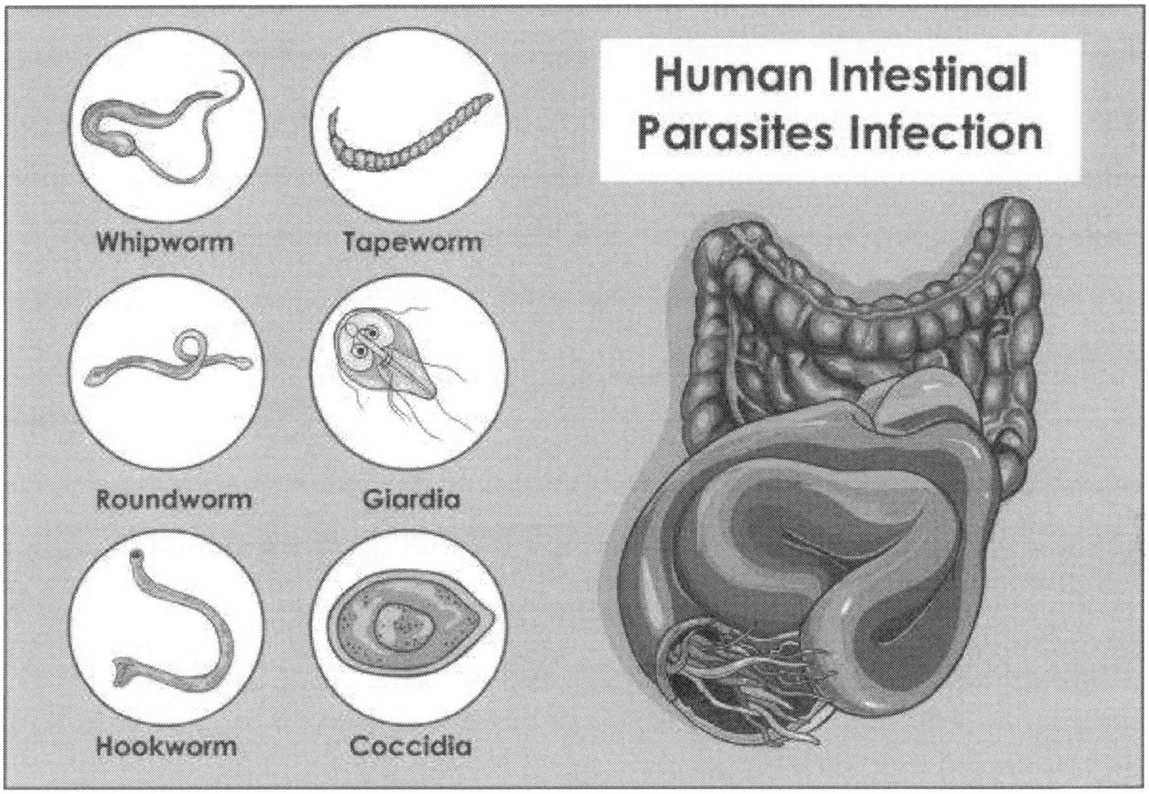

Parasites are a plant or an animal micro-organism that can stay alive in or on another host cell. It gets its nourishment feedings from or on that other micro-organism. Parasitic infections can occur anywhere in tropical and subtropical regions.

There are three main parasitic infections organism that can cause disease in humans. They are:

- Protozoa - a single-celled plasmodium micro-organisms that can survive and multiply inside our body. An example is malaria parasites
- Helminths - a larger and multi-celled micro-organisms that can stay alive inside or outside our body. They are commonly known as worms
- Ecto-parasites - a multi-celled micro-organisms that are able to stay alive on by feeding off on our skin. For example ticks and mosquitos

These diseases can easily spread through the following means:

1) Contaminated soil where it comes in contact with faeces from infected humans or animals.
2) Contaminated drinking water.
3) Contaminated food.

4) Contaminated blood through transfusion from an infected person.
5) Swimming in filthy lakes, rivers and ponds where it comes in contact with Giardia microscopic parasites.
6) Sexual contact with an infected partner.
7) Outdoor cats that happen to come into contact with an infected dead rodents and birds. The infection is then spread through the cat faeces.
8) Insect bites at another infected person which in turn get infected by it.

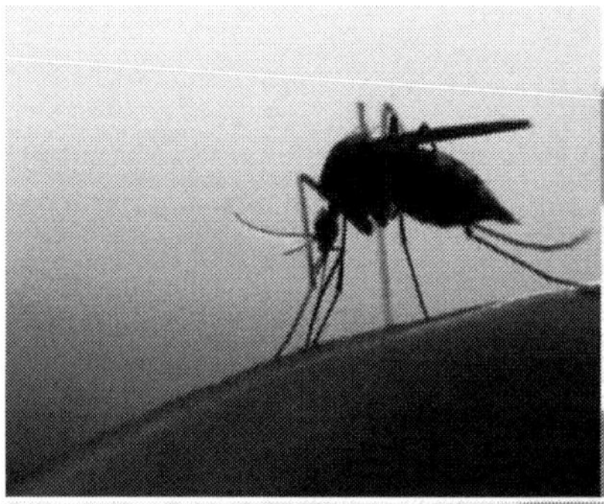
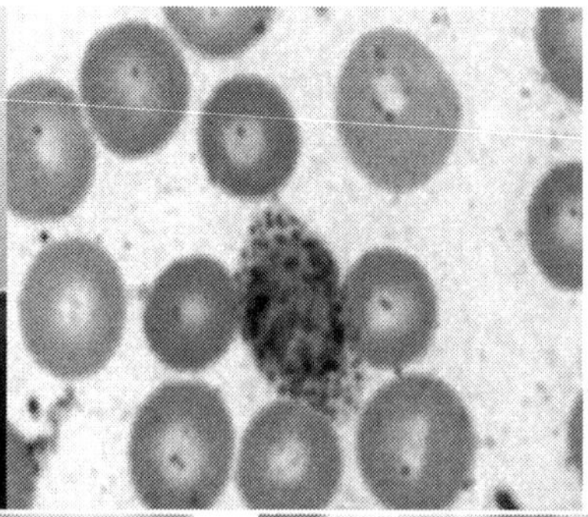
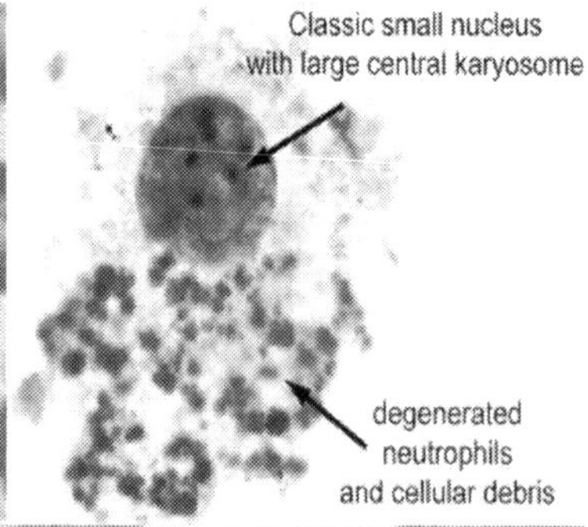

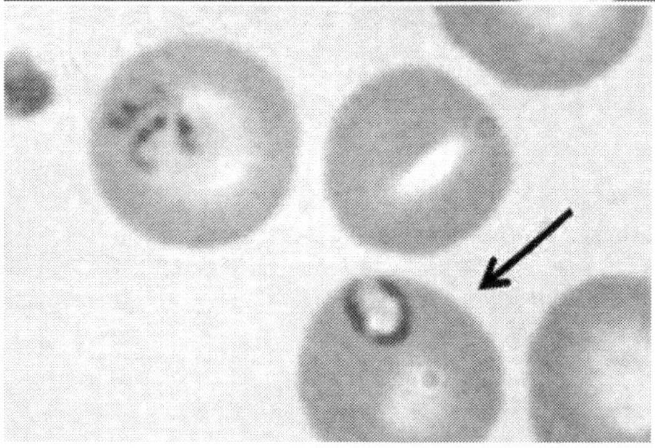
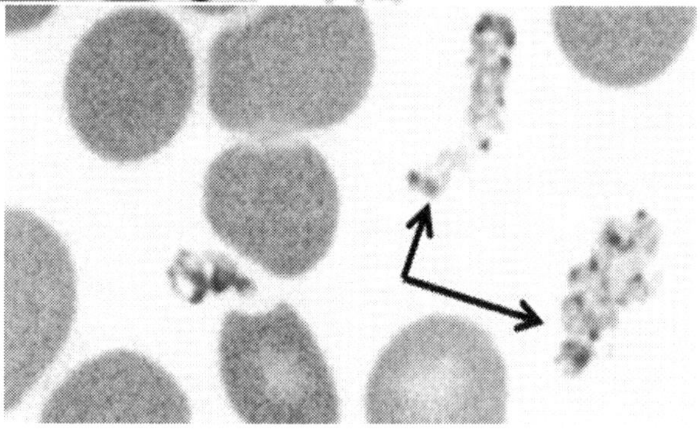

Examples of diseases that can be caused by parasites are Giardiasis, Trichomoniasis, Malaria, Toxoplasmosis, Intestinal worms and Pubic lice.

Some parasitic cases that can get you infected by the following ways:

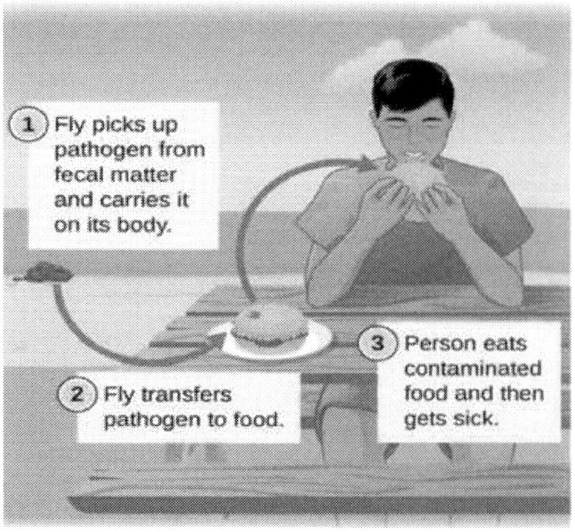

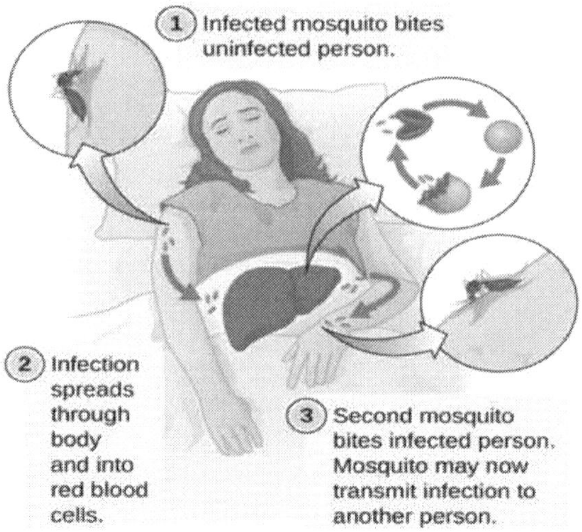

MICROORGANISM FACTS FOR KIDS

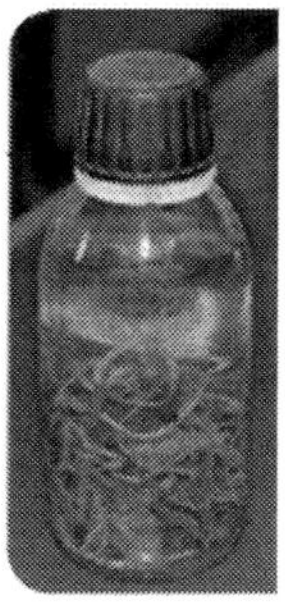

Guinea-worm disease is caused by parasitic worm. They appear to be the largest parasite tissues and commonly affect humans. They usually sneak through the person innermost layer skin tissues to the muscles beneath the skin and cause severe pain especially in and around the joints area. Sufferers will experience high fever, nausea and vomiting. These worms move actively in the water and can live in it for few days.

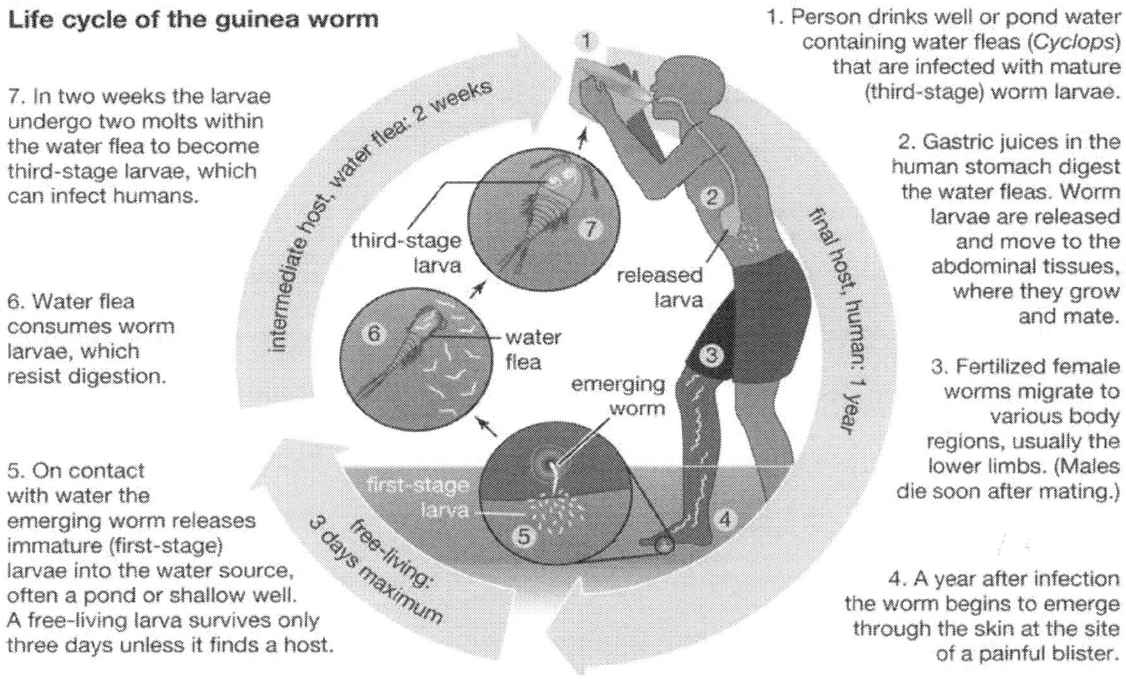

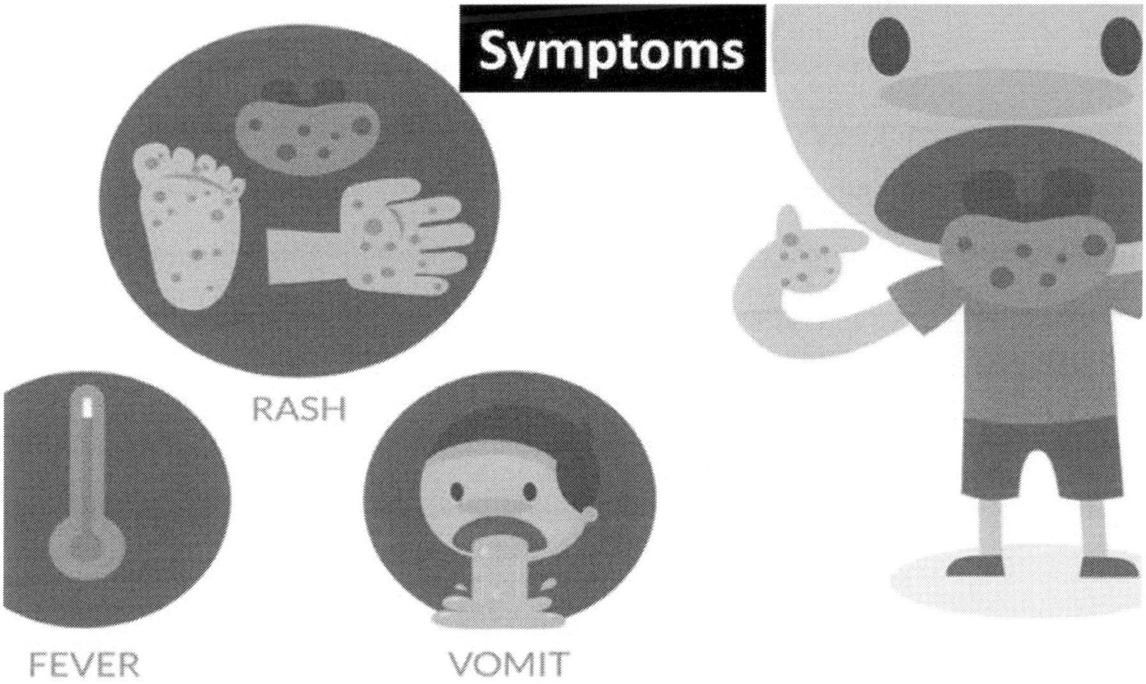

Human Pathogen by Indirect Transmission

Germs can also spread by indirect contact if an infected person touches on a contaminated surface or object unknowingly. For example on a door handles, handrail, table top, or even lift buttons where microorganisms are left behind on the contaminated surface.

Any person who just touched over the contaminated area and then went on to touch the other moist openings area near his eyes, ear, nose or mouth, he will get infected indirectly. The germs sneak in through these openings and find its way to penetrate into his body immune system and attack on the host cells.

There is no 100 percent preventive measures on pathogen transmission in our daily life but the best precaution to minimise such risk of contracting a pathogenic disease is to maintain a good personal hygiene.

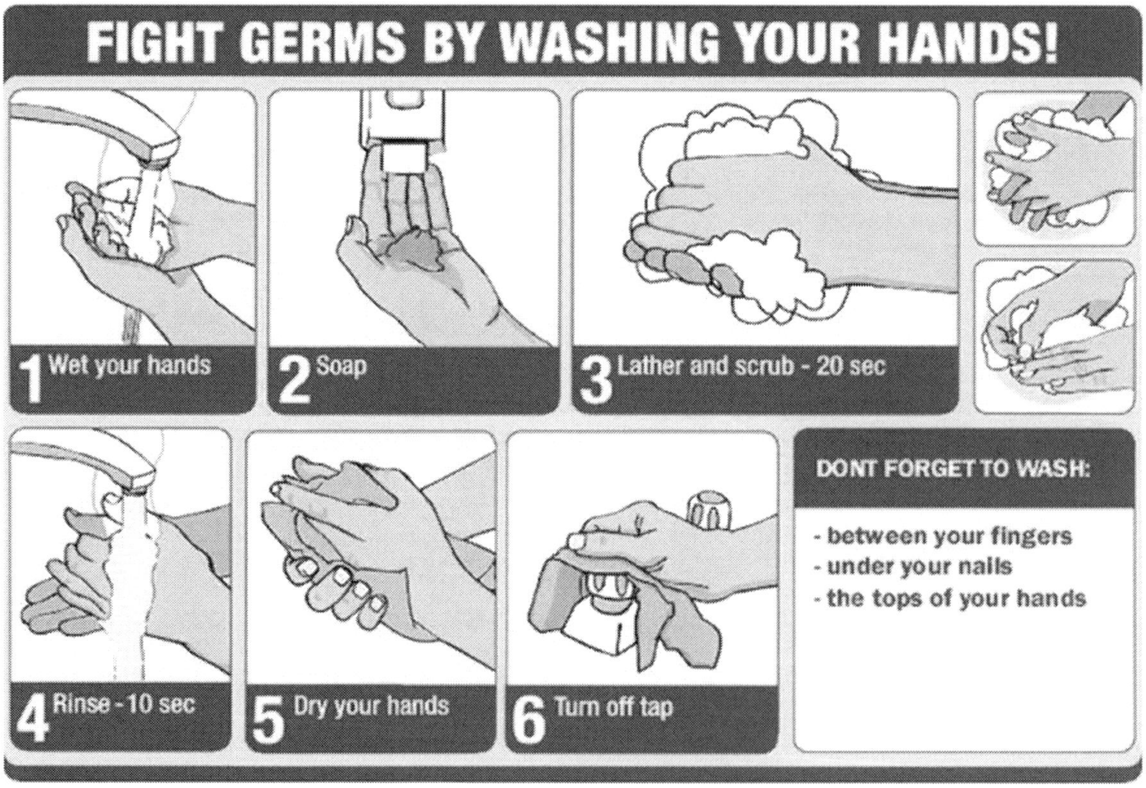

Always remember to wash hands frequently with soap and water after any activities had been carried out. For examples:

1) Going to public restroom.
2) Handling of raw foods.
3) Cleaning up pet and picking up its faeces.

4) When sneezing and coughing, cover nose and mouth to prevent airborne germs transmission. Bin it into proper waste bin after used.

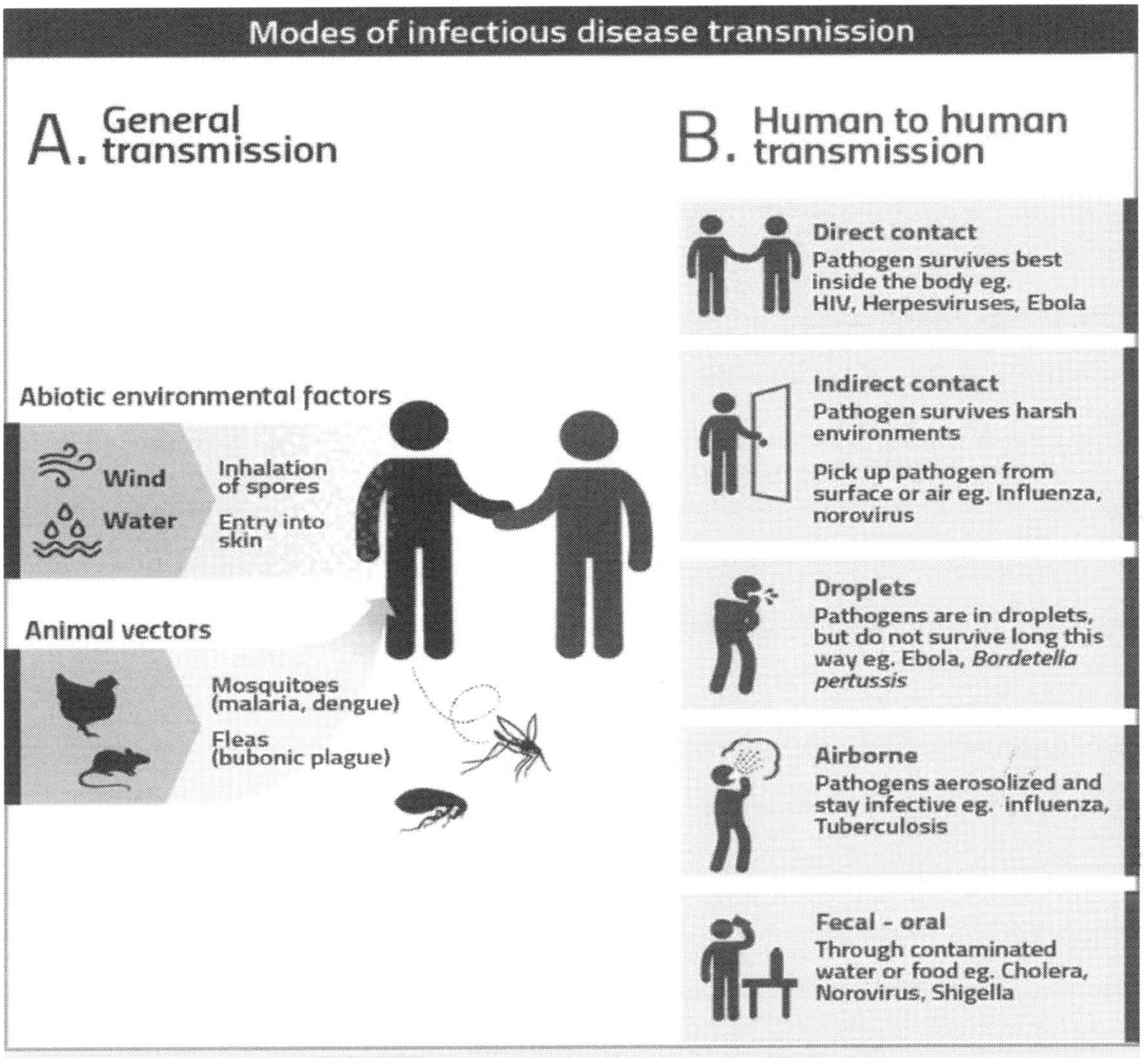

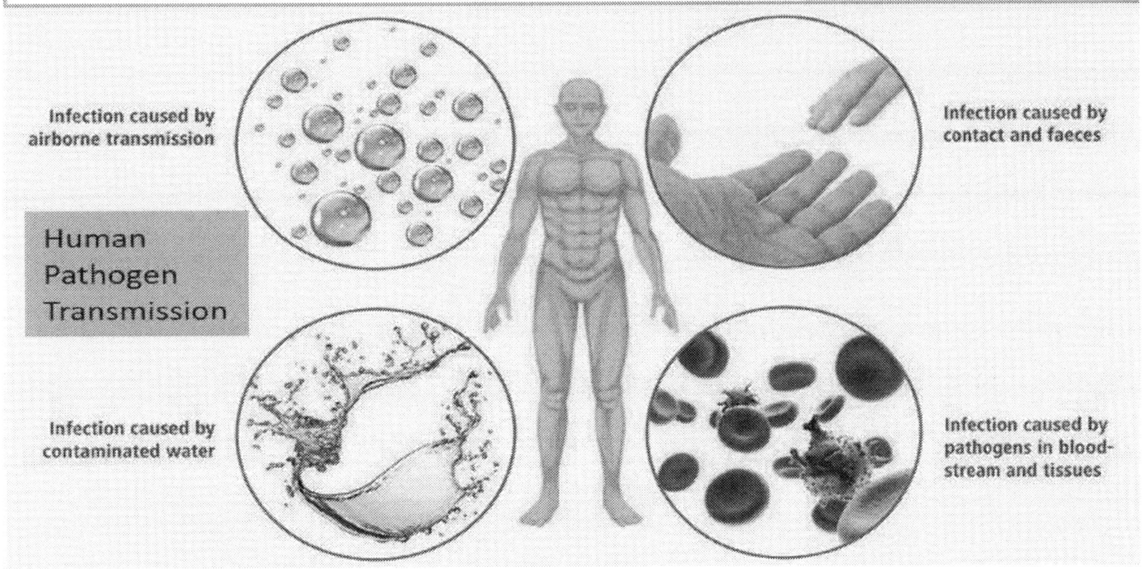

MICROORGANISM FACTS FOR KIDS

Coronavirus Outbreak

This new form of viral pneumonia spreads among the Chinese people in mainland China had already sickened a number of healthcare medical workers. Not only that, it creates confusion, panic and chaos in many parts of the world that had never experienced it before.

From the sharing of important information gathered worldwide, the infection cases keep going up and the numbers keep accumulating day by day without any slowing down of its mean of spread of the infectious virus. It has been widely spread and infected across nationalities, ethnic groups, religions, status and people of all ages across the globe.

Interestingly from the medical studies and evidences on this new virus, COVID-19, children being infected by the virus is still extremely rare and low in figure. Furthermore, it also discovered that in different ethnic group of people, the virus acts differently to their immune response differently.

State news reported that people were seen passing out mysteriously while they were walking in the middle of the streets, taking drinks at local cafe, inside transport cabins, at markets and supermarket stores etc. in some countries. All the related cases were seen to experience some difficulties in grasping air for breathing which look like the coronavirus symptoms.

As death tolls and coronavirus infections continue to spiral upwards uncontrollably, World Health Organisation officially make an announcement to the world public health emergency a global **"Pandemic"** alert warnings on 30 Jan 2020. The following day, America also make its stand towards her health emergency preparedness announcement. Preventive measures were outlaid gradually in phases to get its people protected from the coronavirus pandemic.

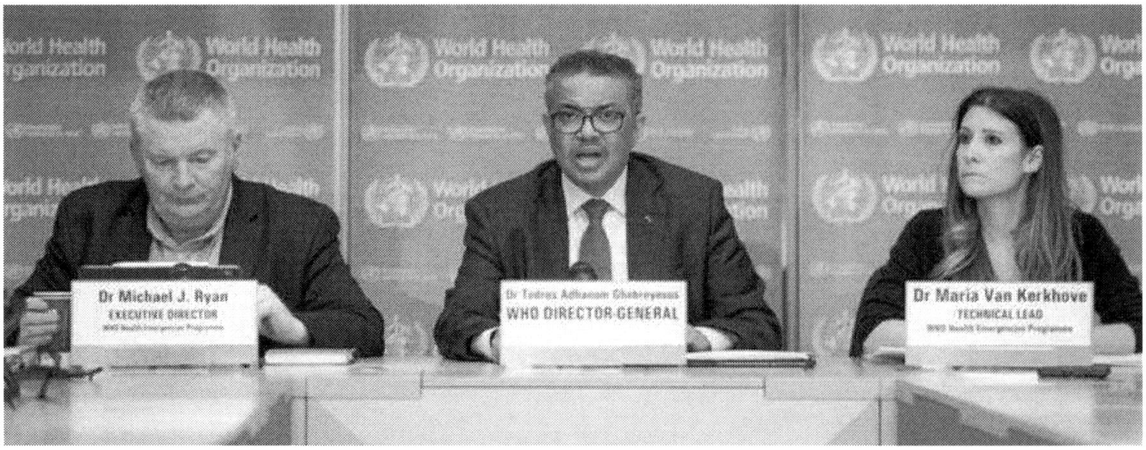

MICROORGANISM FACTS FOR KIDS

Pandemic Alert

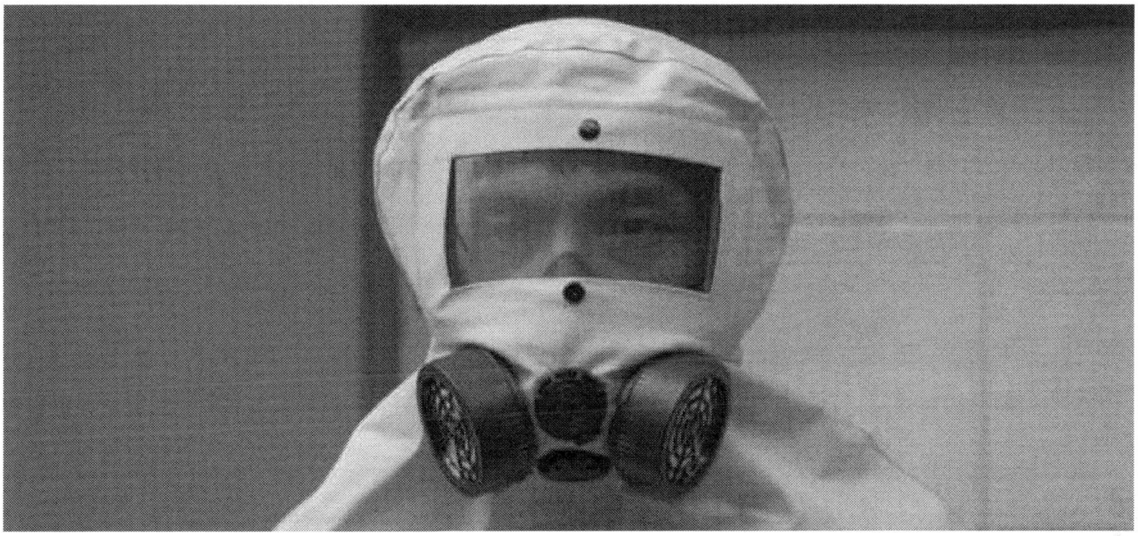

Pandemic outbreak derived from epidemic situation where there was an **exponentially steep rising of infection cases** were seen to be rapidly spreading from **one continent to another** across the nation, affecting quite a large group of people being infected from person-to-person at the same time and causing more deaths than the epidemic outbreak. Examples of devastating pandemics outbreak situation are:

1. 1918 Spanish flu (H1N1 virus) outbreak which had seen taking away 50 million lives worldwide during the influenza season
2. Influenza type A (H3N2) virus outbreak in 1968 saw a million people deaths worldwide
3. Swine flu virus outbreak in 2009 saw hundreds of thousands of people death
4. AIDS and TB diseases
5. And now this new virus, COVID-19, outbreak had swept across more than 16 million confirmed cases worldwide to-date. This figure is not going to stop there until there is a vaccine developed as early as possible to treat those infected and to control the situation.

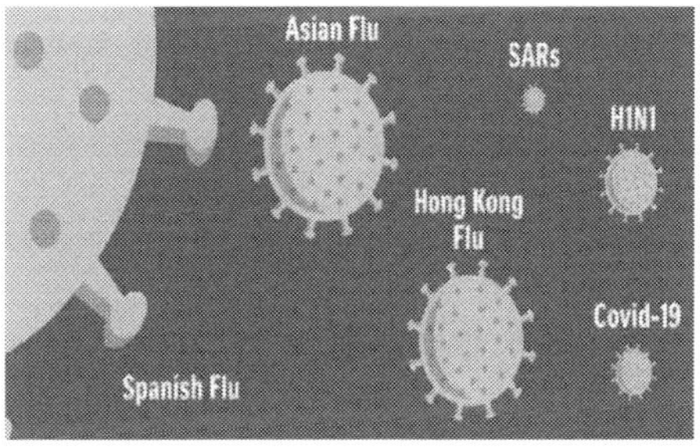

People with pre-existing and underlying health medical conditions such as diabetes, chronic heart diseases and hypertension symptoms are more vulnerable and prone to get infected easily from this infectious virus. It is advisable to stay indoors and restrict their outside movement to keep safe during this health crisis situation for their own good.

MICROORGANISM FACTS FOR KIDS

Epidemic Outbreak Crisis

Epidemic outbreak occurred when there was a widespread diseases that were spinning out of control, but **at a stable containment by infected people among one or more communities within a geographic location** inside a country boundaries.

Examples of epidemics outbreak situation are:

1) Natural disaster
    - Tropical Storms
    - Floods
    - Earthquakes
    - Droughts
2) Disease outbreak such as
    - Ebola virus disease (Ebola haemorrhagic fever) in West Africa claimed 11,300 lives between year 2013 and 2016.
      The strains of the virus could cause severe illness in humans, animals and even death.
    - SARS-CoV outbreak in 2003 claimed 800 deaths in Africa.
    - MERS-CoV outbreak in 2012 from Middle East was originated in Saudi Arabia.

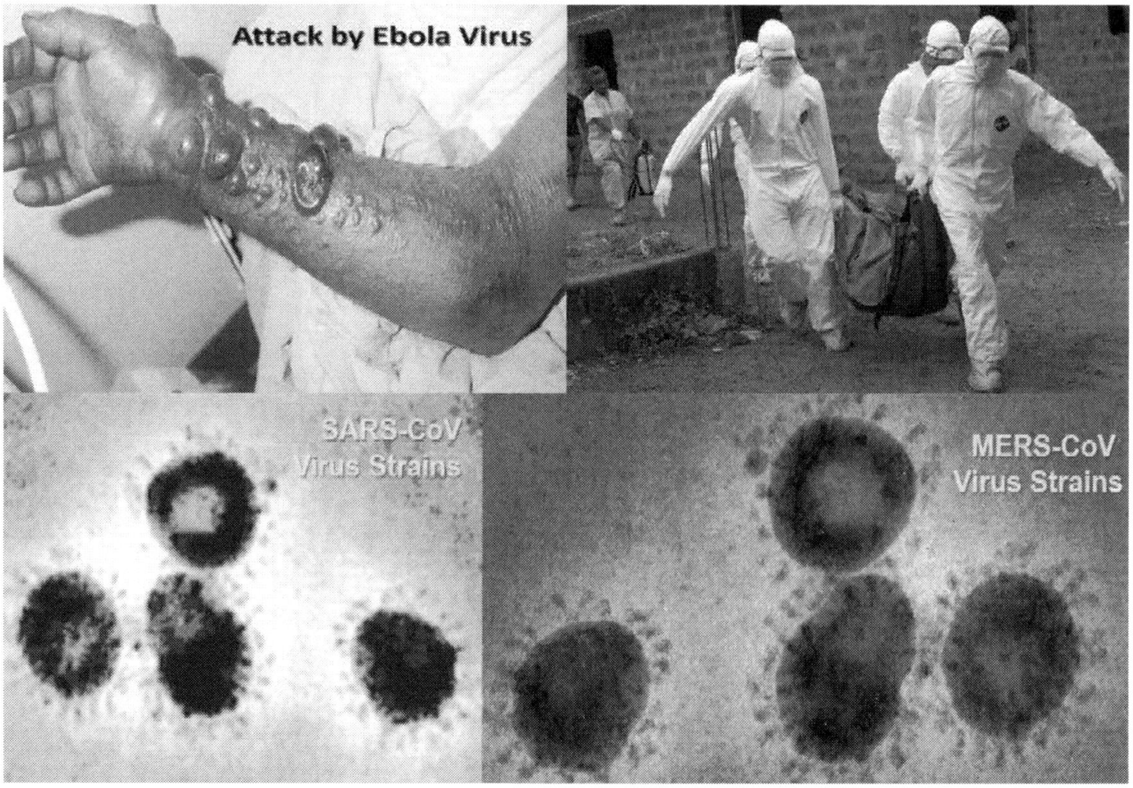

Microorganism Facts For Kids

The coronavirus family cover a wide scope of viruses that can behave simply a cold-like symptoms from a common cold illnesses to severe diseases such as MERS-Cov, **M**iddle **E**ast **R**espiratory **S**yndrome, and SARS-Cov, **S**evere **A**cute **R**espiratory **S**yndrome, and now with the inclusive of this new COVID-19, **CO**rono**V**irus **D**isease 20**19**, virus strains.

The disease can transmit between animals and humans, and vice versa. The only main difference in COVID-19 infections can be seen by a number of unlinked cases being infected with this disease by asymptomatic person who are positive carrier does not inhibit any physical symptoms which is harder to trace its whereabouts.

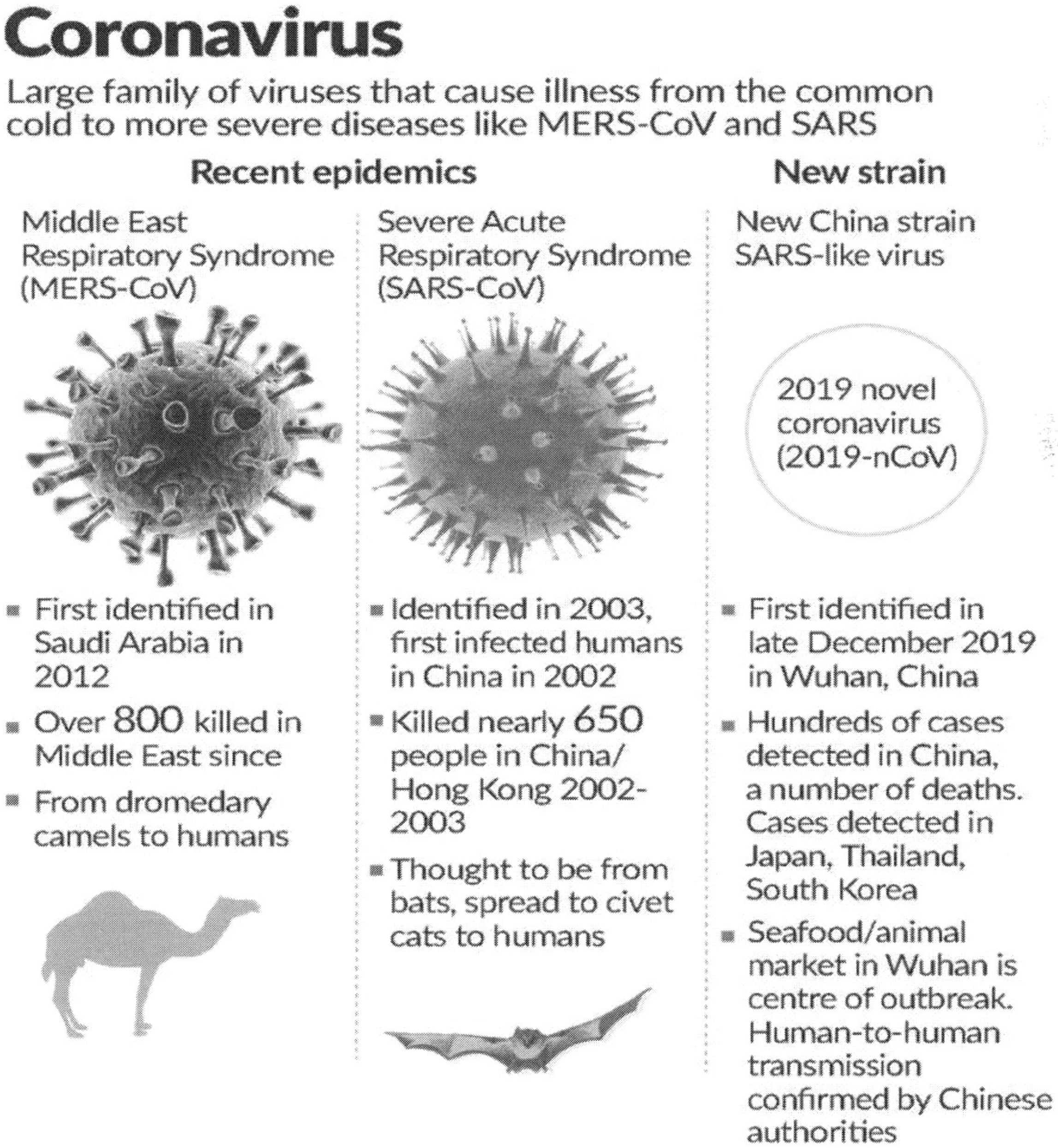

Microorganism Facts For Kids

Endemic Outbreak Crisis

An endemic outbreak happens when there is an infection within a certain area, or population in a specific geographic region.

Endemics outbreak can arise from:

1) Cholera - It is a bacterial disease that can give rise to severe diarrhoea and dehydration in human body. It normally spread by contaminated water. Those infected will show the symptoms around 2-3 days later.
2) Malaria disease is spread by Aedes mosquitoes. People who get bites from these mosquitoes will get infected and symptoms will show up around a week time.
3) Chickenpox is commonly spread in young children.

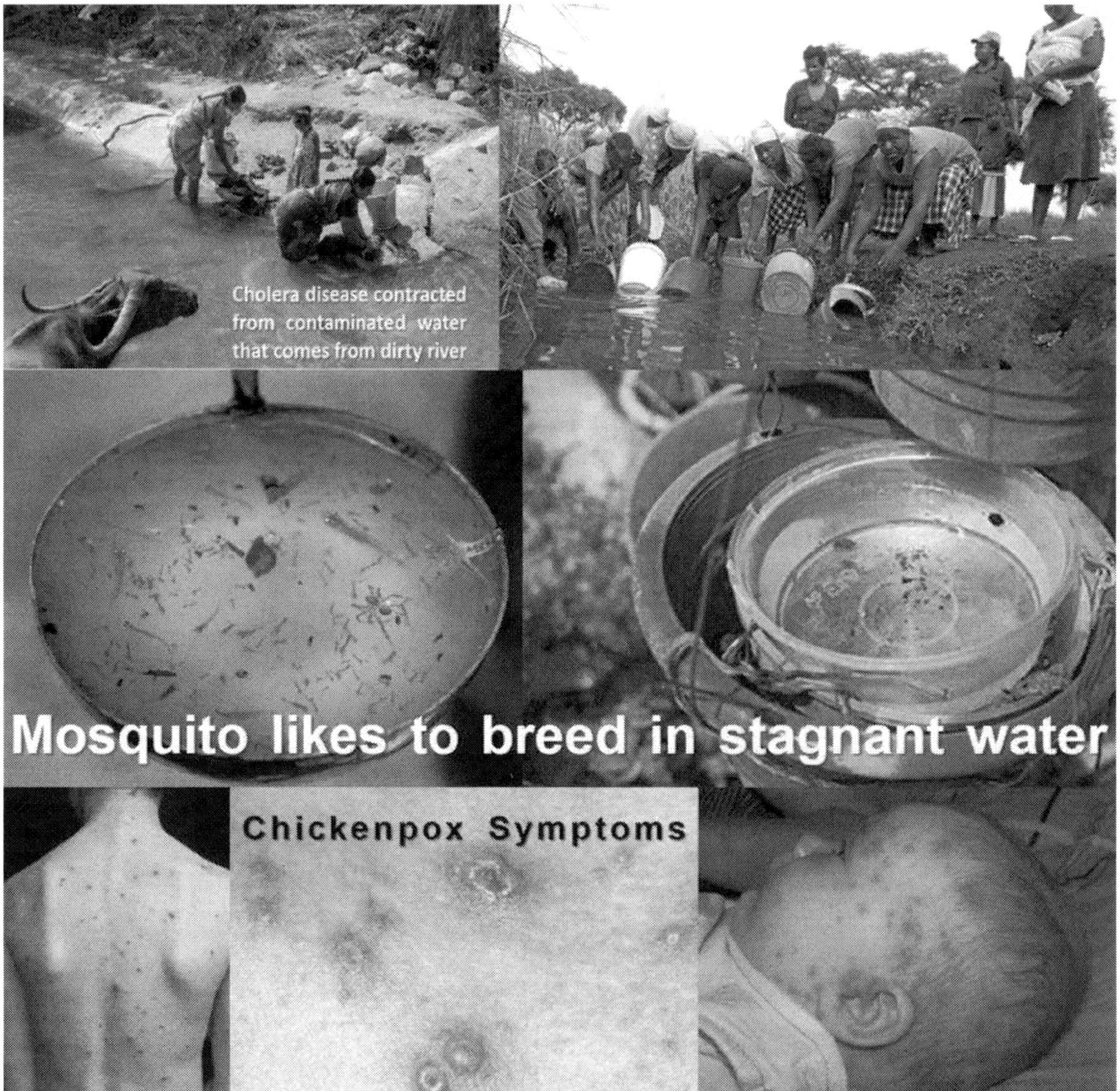
Cholera disease contracted from contaminated water that comes from dirty river
Mosquito likes to breed in stagnant water
Chickenpox Symptoms

Outbreak Crisis

An outbreak crisis can arise when there is a new, contagious and infectious germ disease that begins to infect the whole population.

Swift preventive measures need to put up fast to control and prevent its infections from further spreading within a community or across the world. Such a crisis typically can last weeks or even couple of years.

Virus outbreak transmissions can infect person-to-person, animal-to-person contacts or can from the environment situation.

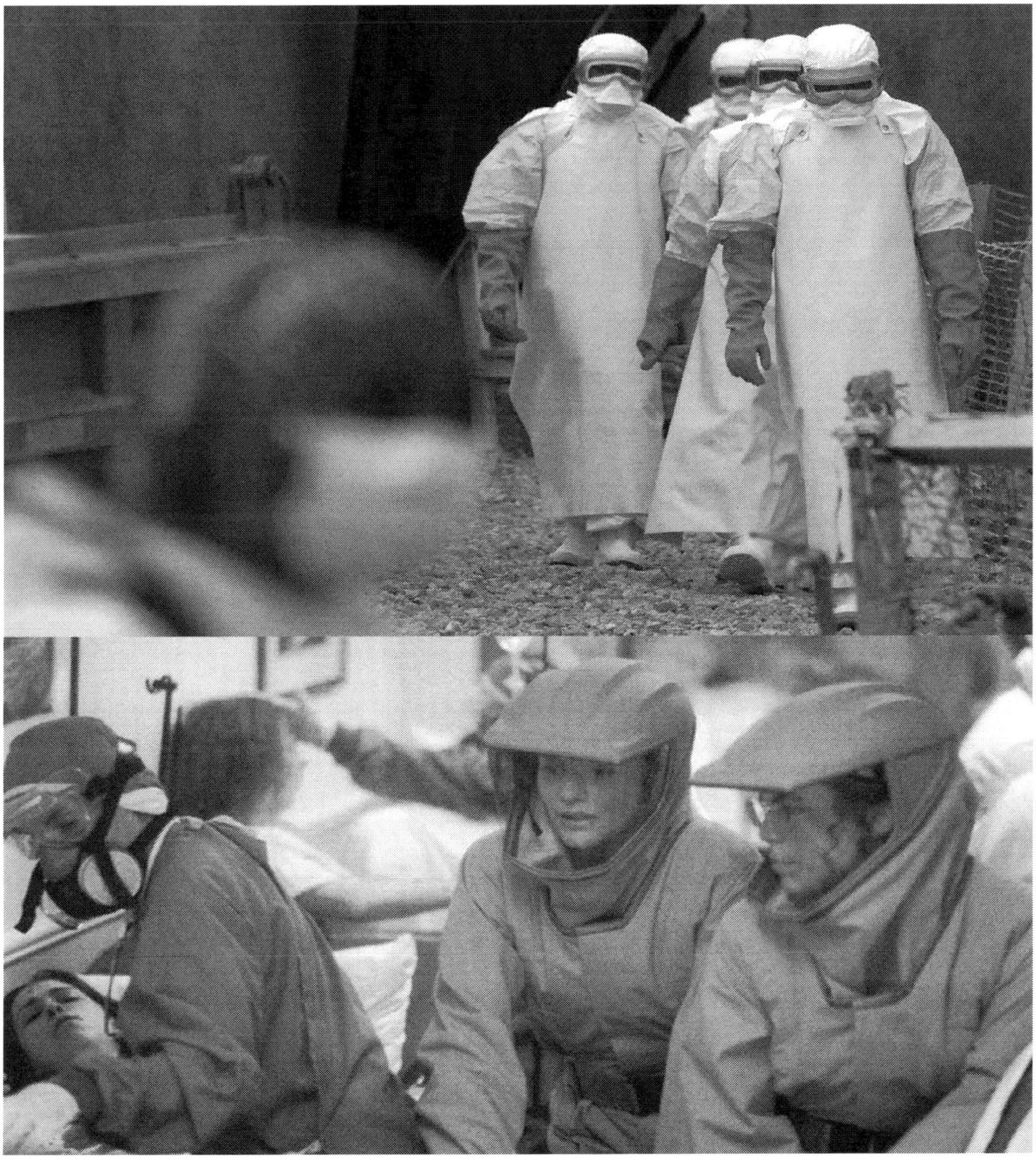

MICROORGANISM FACTS FOR KIDS

Diseases

A disease is an abnormal condition that can affect a living organism with an onset symptoms. The disease can slowly spread to other bodily parts or to the entire body.

Physical symptoms of the disease give rise to emotional symptoms but some can severely affect the nervous system.

Categories of diseases include bacterial, blood, autoimmune, cancer, digestive, heart, nerve, sexually transmitted and thyroid. Viruses or bacterial infections are diseases that can continually present symptomatically.

Prevention of diseases is possible only if ones takes good care of hygiene seriously, including proper sanitation, proper nutrition, frequent exercise and vaccination.

Diseases can be classified as Infectious and Non-infectious types.

- Infectious diseases - Viruses that are communicable and can easily catch from coming near to infected person through airborne germs transmission by direct and indirect contacts. Common infectious diseases are Colds, Influenza, Measles, Mumps, Tuberculosis, Pneumonia, Smallpox etc.
- Non-infectious diseases are Asthma, Cancer and Arthritis.

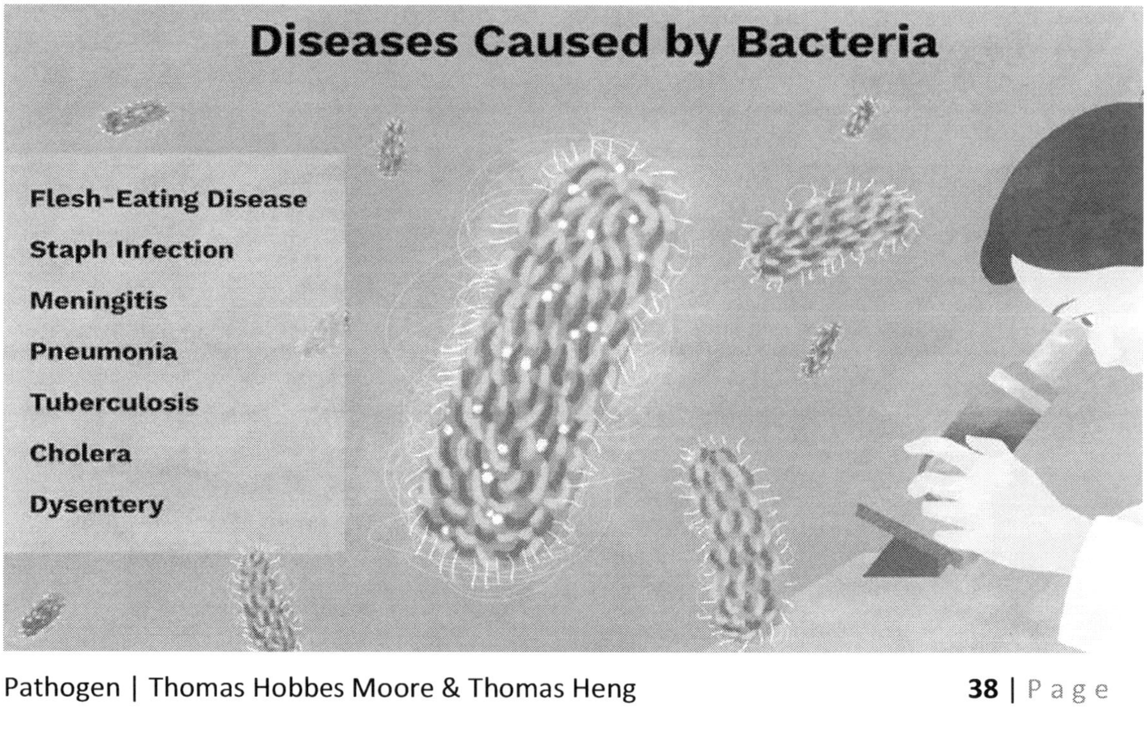

MICROORGANISM FACTS FOR KIDS

Appropriate Precautions for COVID-19 disease

Adhere to the advice given by local health authority to protect yourself and others by knowing and understanding the factual of the coronavirus disease. Take responsibility and appropriate precautions to fight against this new virus as we move to curb it until a vaccine is developed.

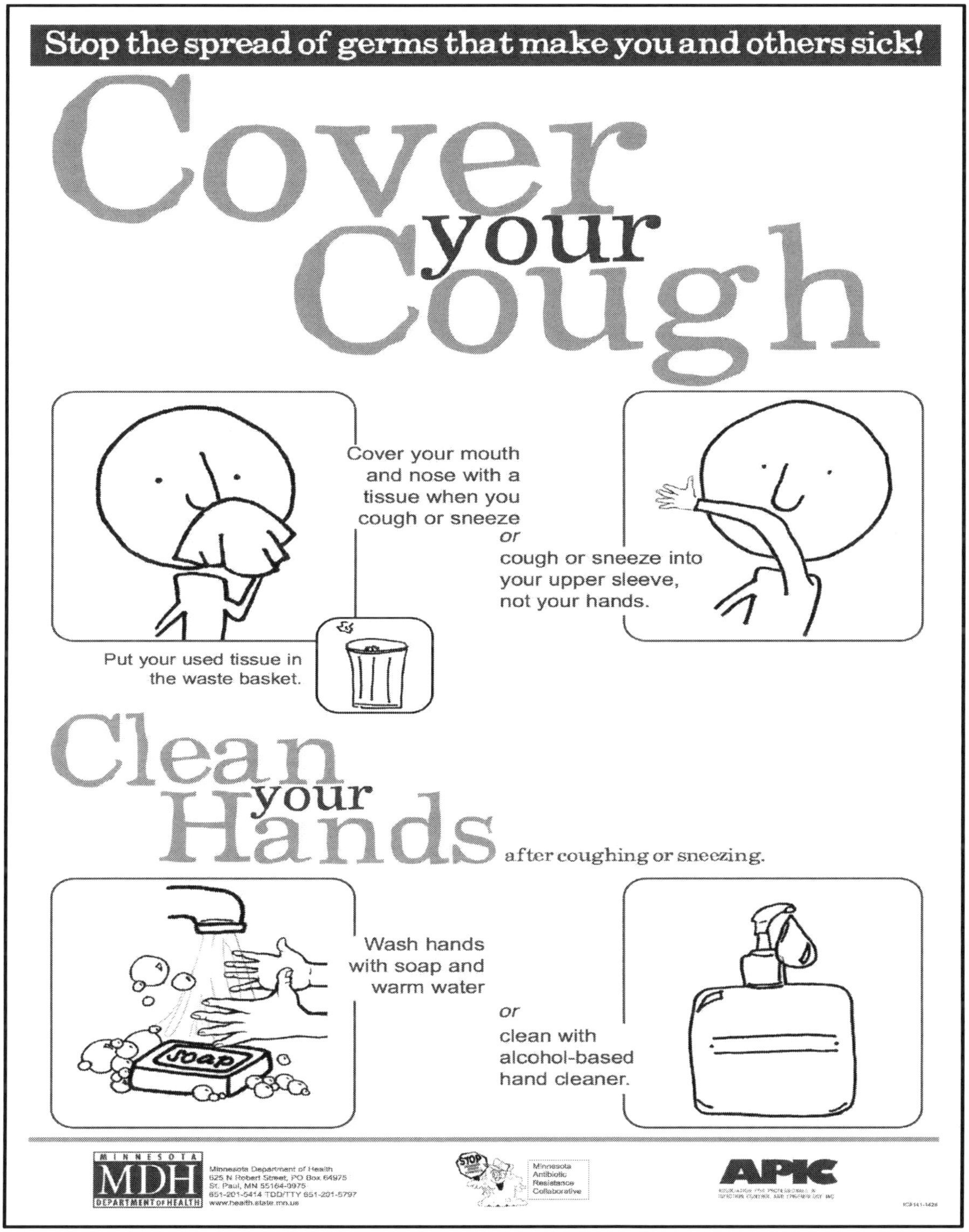

MICROORGANISM FACTS FOR KIDS

Germs and UVC Rays

Germs pandemic behaviour doesn't care about seasonal patterns evolving from the starting cause to the viral outbreaks.

For example Spanish flu can be peaked at summer month's period while seasonal influenza peaks at winter time.

Sunlight comprises of three kinds of UV rays, namely:

1. UVA
2. UVB
3. UVC

Except UVC ray, both UVA and UVB rays can be quite damaging and harmful to human skins. Light spectrum from UVC rays which consist of shorter and energetic wavelengths can apply to areas where it can effectively use to destroy genetically viral microbes swiftly.

Artificial UVC equipment offers a staple sterilisation method of sweeping and killing off these living microorganisms that thrive on surfaces.

Artificial UVC mobile robots are rolling out to places such as healthcare, aviation, offices and factories, and transport sectors to help decontaminate the surrounding environment.

Some parasites are resistant to chemical disinfectants like chlorine. Only by using UVC method, they can be totally eradicated. It serves as a failsafe alternative.

1. UVC-Emitting Mobile Robots deploy in hospital environments

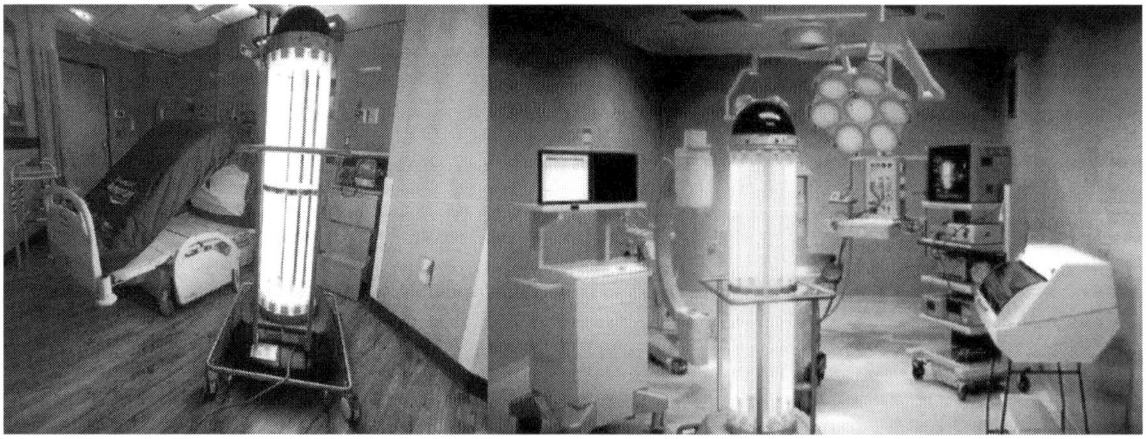

Robots are using UVC blue light beams, glowing like light sabres, to zap hospital viruses in patient rooms, operating theatres, cleaning floors etc.

MICROORGANISM FACTS FOR KIDS

1. Bus disinfection by using UVC lights in public transportation

Alert!

Stern warning, aware the potential dangers of the UVC, Ultraviolet-C light.

- NEVER shine on human skins or use it to sterilise hands as these can cause skin irritations. It is one of the major causes in skin cancer.
- Stay at least 5 metres apart from the harmful UVC light when in use.

UV chambers are set up in huge cleaning room. Then, remotely controlling the cleaning process through the 210 UV tubes by passing the UV light on the bus interiors and exteriors as a way of disinfection process.

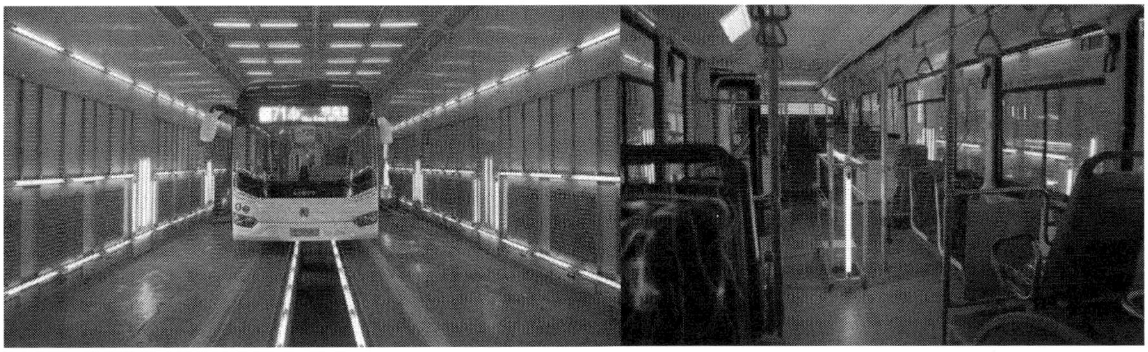

2. Banknotes disinfection employs by banks

Central bank is relying on UVC technology to disinfect all contaminated paper monies.

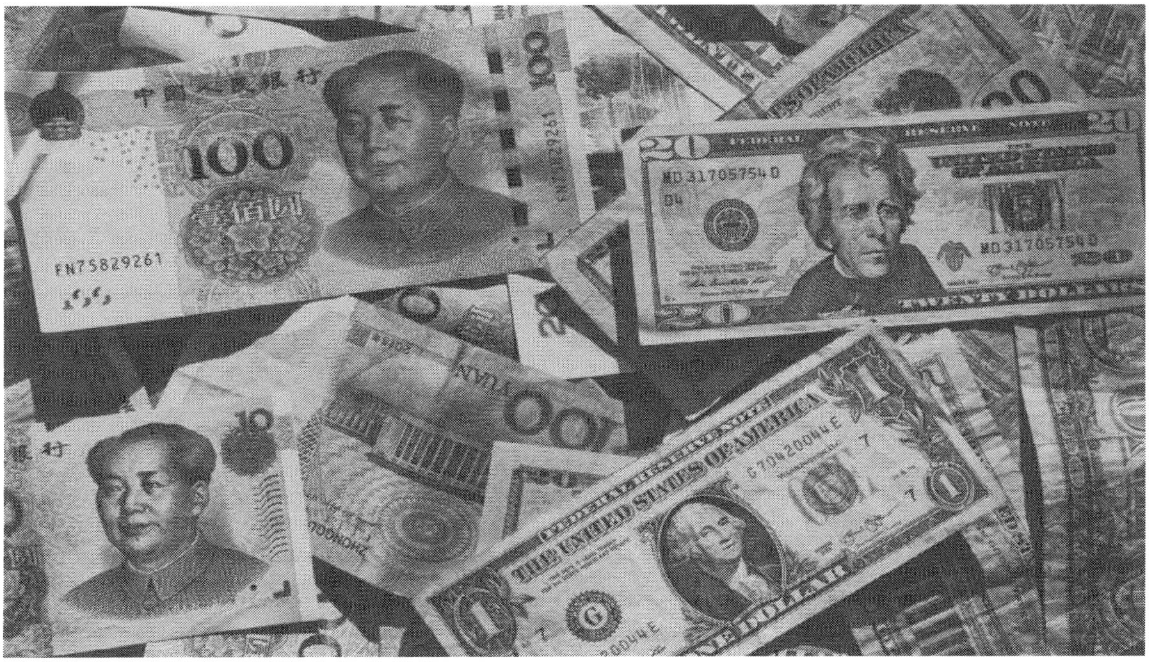

MICROORGANISM FACTS FOR KIDS

Germs and Temperatures

Bacteria Survival Information

Germs spread person to person and contaminate equipment or surfaces if infected person left its contaminated particles behind it.

1. Bacteria cannot multiply Itself but stay dormant at below temperature 32^0F (0^0C).
2. Bacteria multiply slowly when temperature is in the range between 32^0 and 40^0F (0^0C-6^0C).
3. Danger Zone when bacteria can multiply rapidly when temperature hits the range between 40^0 and 140^0F (4^0C-60^0C).
4. Bacteria stop to multiply by itself and start to die off when temperature hits the range between 140^0 and 165^0F (60^0C-74^0C).
5. Bacteria will be totally eradicated if temperature hits above 212^0F (100^0C).

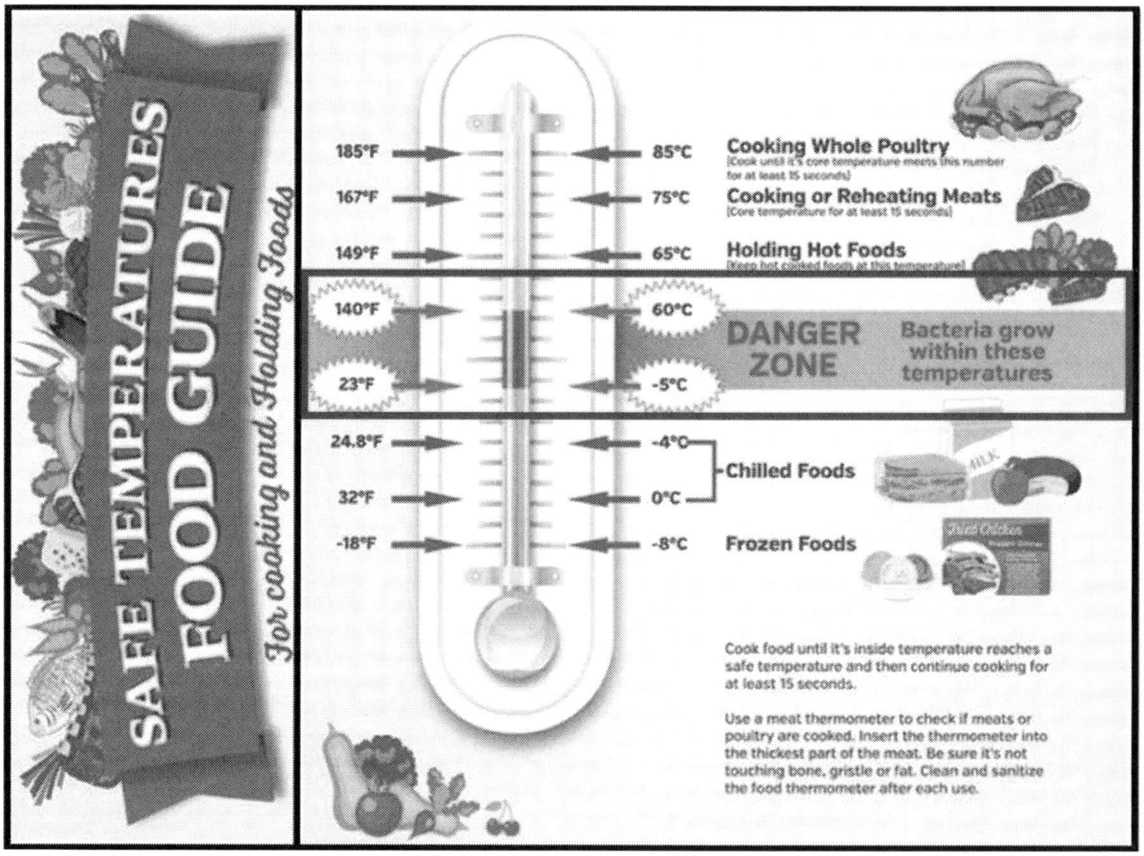

Hot temperatures at above 140^oF (60^oC) can kill germs instantly. Freezing temperatures do not kill germs but rather it makes them stay dormant until they are thawed, and gradually inured to higher cooking temperatures.

Laundry

Germs can spread via clothes.

Washing clothes at 30°C temperature is not enough to kill germs. It is even likely to spread germs instead.

Clothes need to wash in lukewarm water and dried at temperatures at around 140°F (>60°C) to kill many microorganisms.

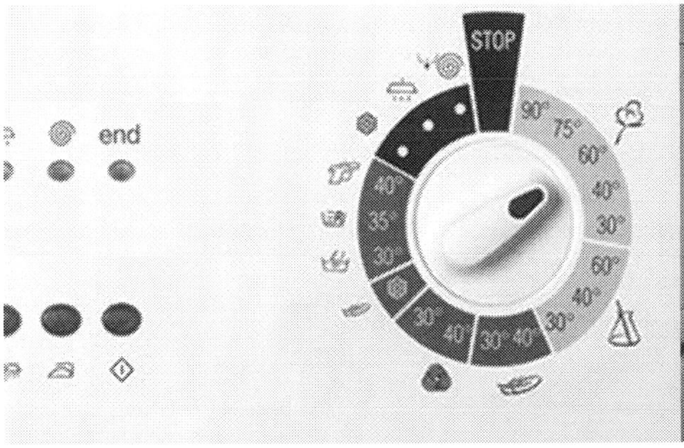

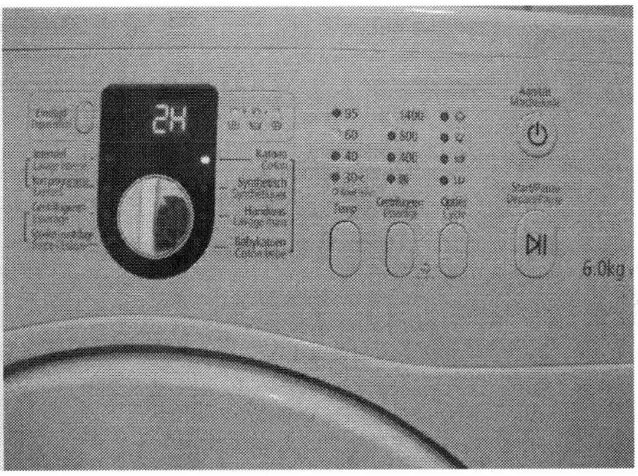

Contaminated Surfaces

Inside our house, the likely areas that can easily infect by germs are in the kitchen and toilet areas.

To prevent germs, use soap and water to wash our hands.

Use disinfectant liquid like Dettol to clean kitchen and household surfaces. Pouring some disinfectant liquid and mix with flooring cleaning agent to kill germs.

Chopping board must keep dry as dampness can make germs thrive and continue to multiply itself.

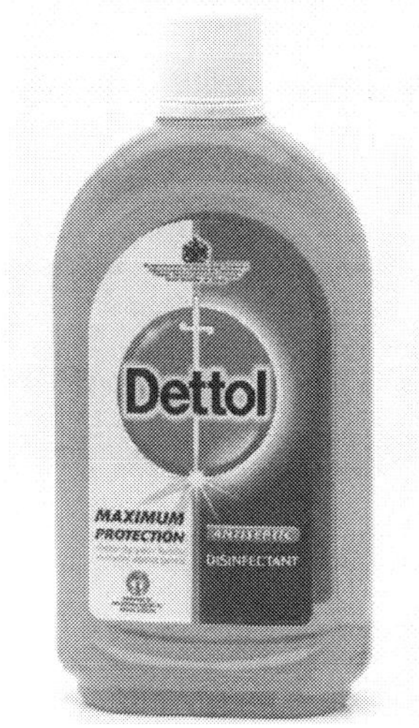

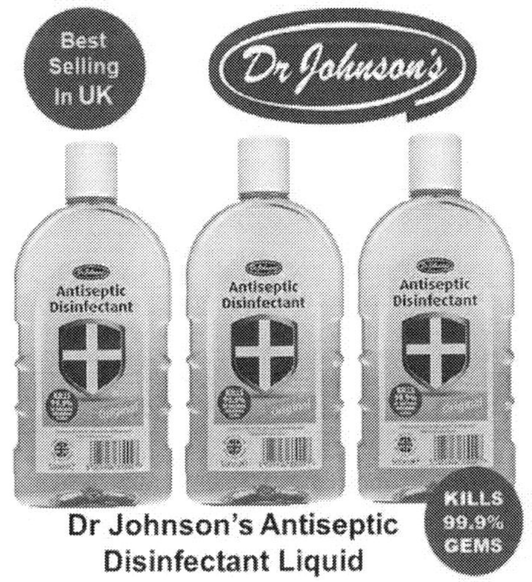

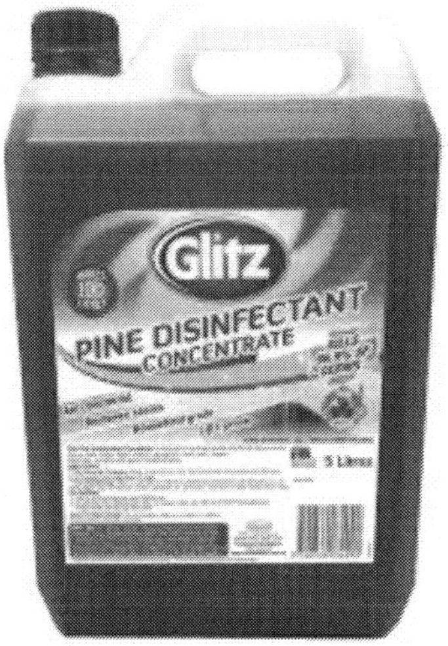

Microorganism Facts For Kids

Food Safety Advice

Unless you need to prepare food within a short period of time or otherwise when putting food outside at temperatures between 40° and 140°F, you are actually putting and exposing the food bacteria invasion.

Food contamination usually occurs when food is left untouched for more than 2 hours. By then, it is considered unsafe to consume.

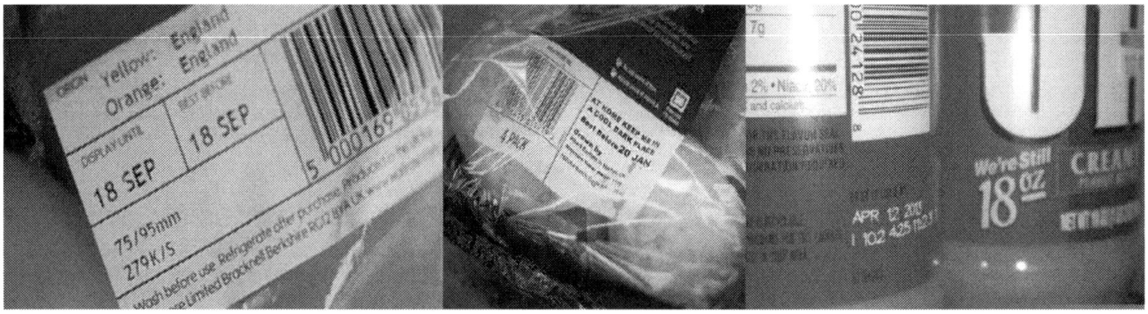

Food Hygiene Rules

1. Do not eat expired food. Always consume food by the “used-by” date found on the food label sticker.
2. Cook food thoroughly. Especially meat, it must be well cooked until the meat is no longer pinkish in colour.
3. Store raw meat, poultry and seafood at the freezer and not the fridge compartment area.
4. Avoid neither putting raw meat, poultry and fish together with other vegetables nor washing them together as these give rise to food cross-contamination.

   Bacteria can easily spread from raw meats to other foods, cooking surface and utensils when hygiene process of preparing has been overlooked in this manner.

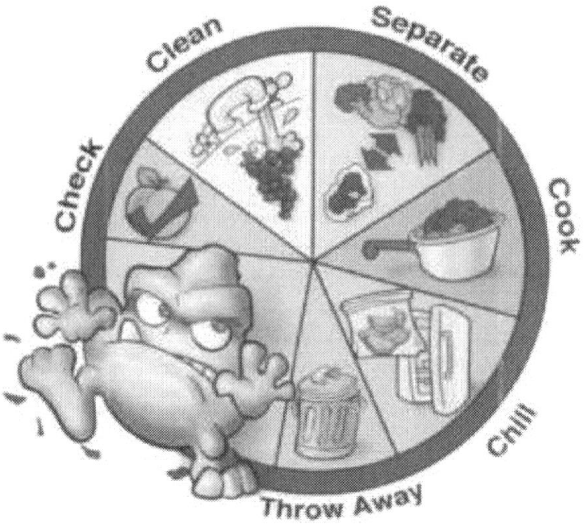

Microorganism Facts For Kids

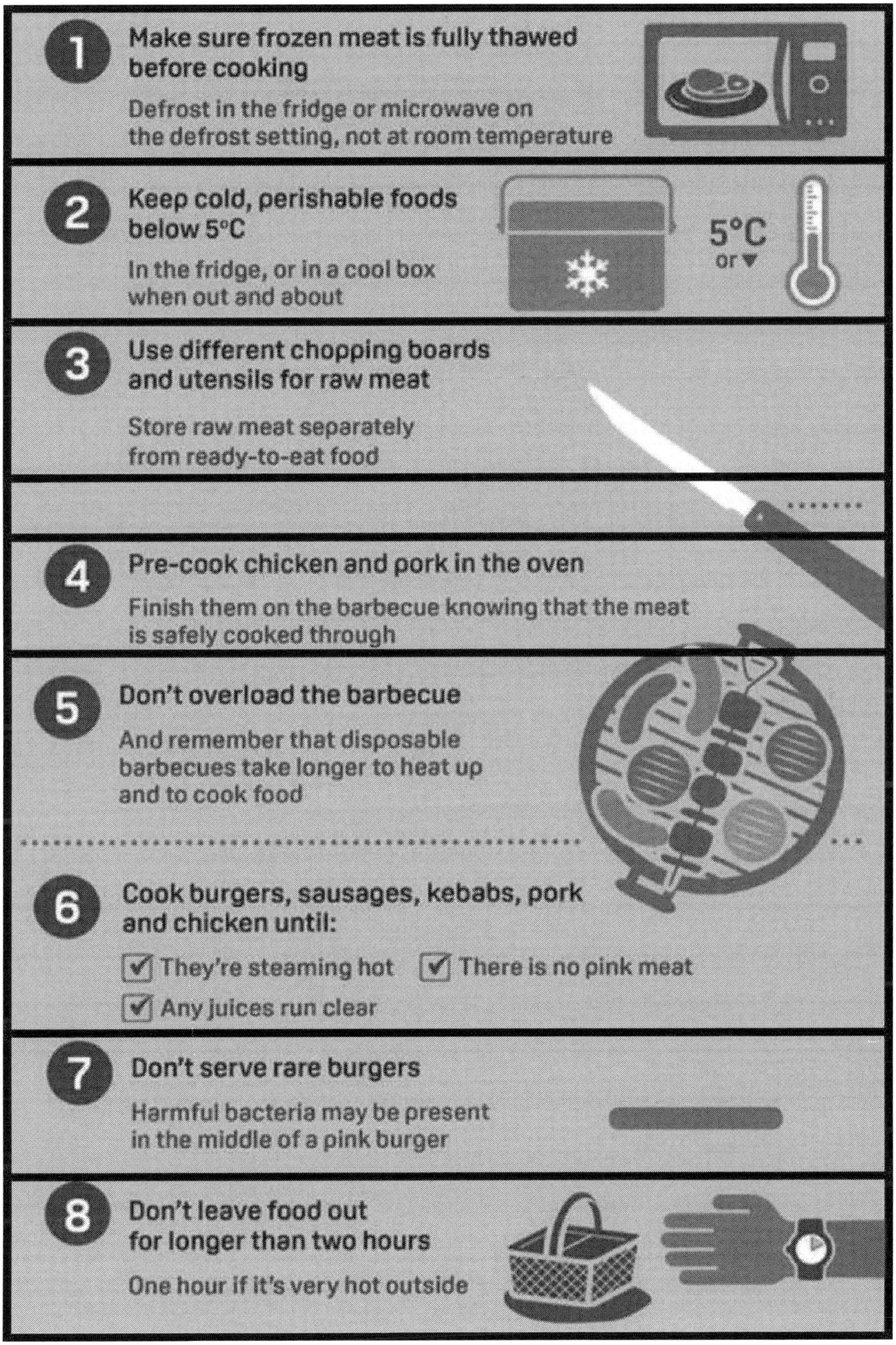

Wildlife Trade and Global Disease Emergence

Wildlife animals trade usually involve in killing animals like tigers, leopards and crocodiles for its skins to make into leisurely goods and souvenirs, consumption for food delicacy, medicinal usage, elephant ivories for ornaments and some sold as pets. This illegal trade of exotic wildlife is rapidly growing in the world and reaping in billions of dollar businesses.

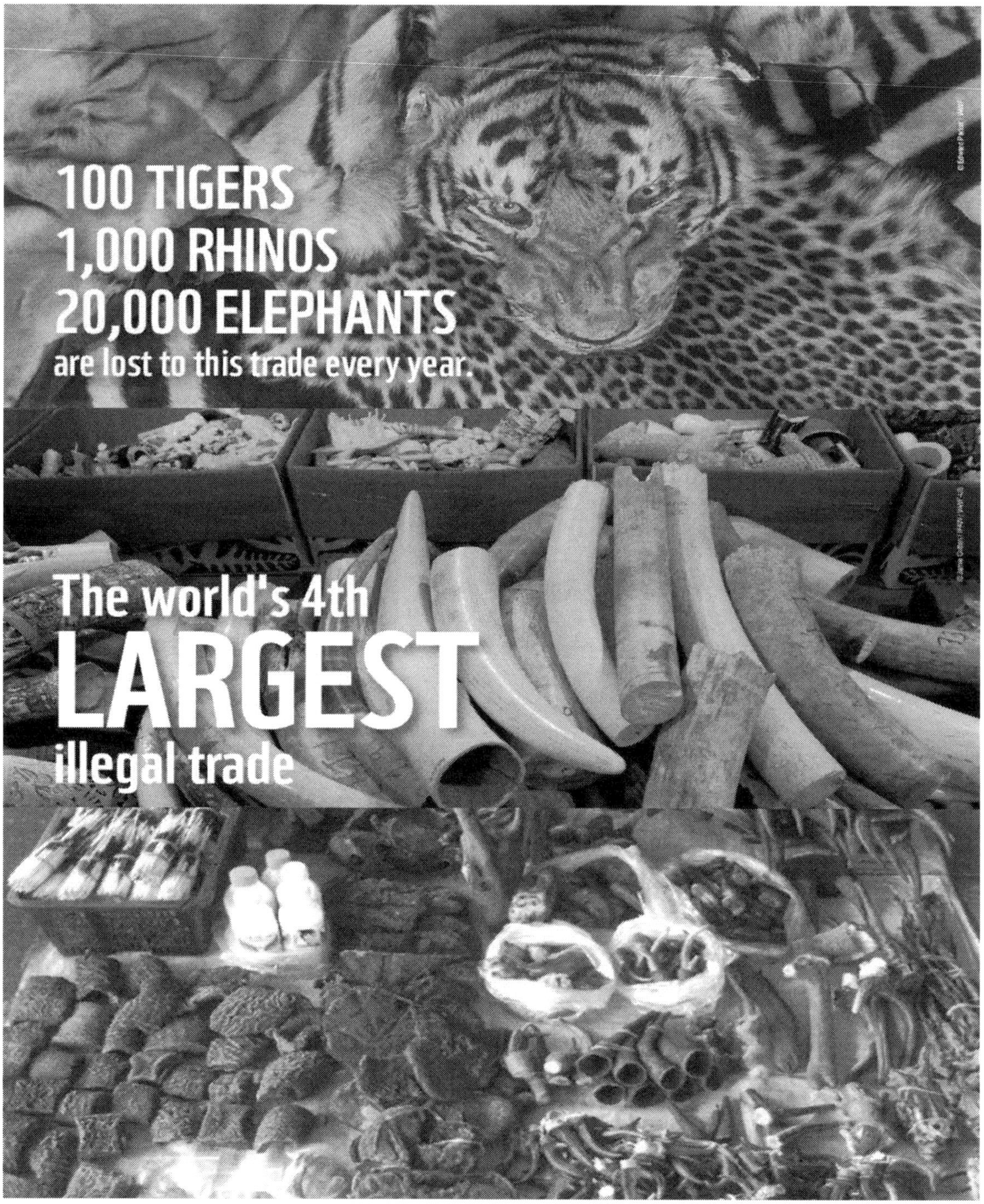
100 TIGERS
1,000 RHINOS
20,000 ELEPHANTS
are lost to this trade every year.
The world's 4th
LARGEST
illegal trade

MICROORGANISM FACTS FOR KIDS

Global trade of exotic wildlife on the other hand can also induce the emergence of diseases associated with it. It can spark a potential human health risks. Virus strains can be transported from exporting regions or during transits and can cause jump species' barriers into humans, infecting those who are in close proximity with it.

These wildlife-borne diseases bring in an increased risk of unchecked pathogens, contributing to the emergence of new diseases in livestock which can transmit lethal infectious diseases through human-animal interactions inherent in the global wildlife trade.

Studies conducted and shared by US Centers for Disease Control and Prevention (CDC) had scientific evidences to prove that pathogens such as zoonotic retroviruses, simian foamy viruses and primate herpes viruses were all originated from the illegal livestocks. Moreover, those experiments conducted over the confiscated livestocks brought in for laboratory investigations had established the factual and traceability of the diseases linked with these illegal wildlife trades.

Wildlife illegal trading can create a serious impact on our ecosystems after their habitat loss, a threat to the extinction of endangered species to serious disturbances in their jungle life. For examples white elephants, rhinos, pangolins etc.

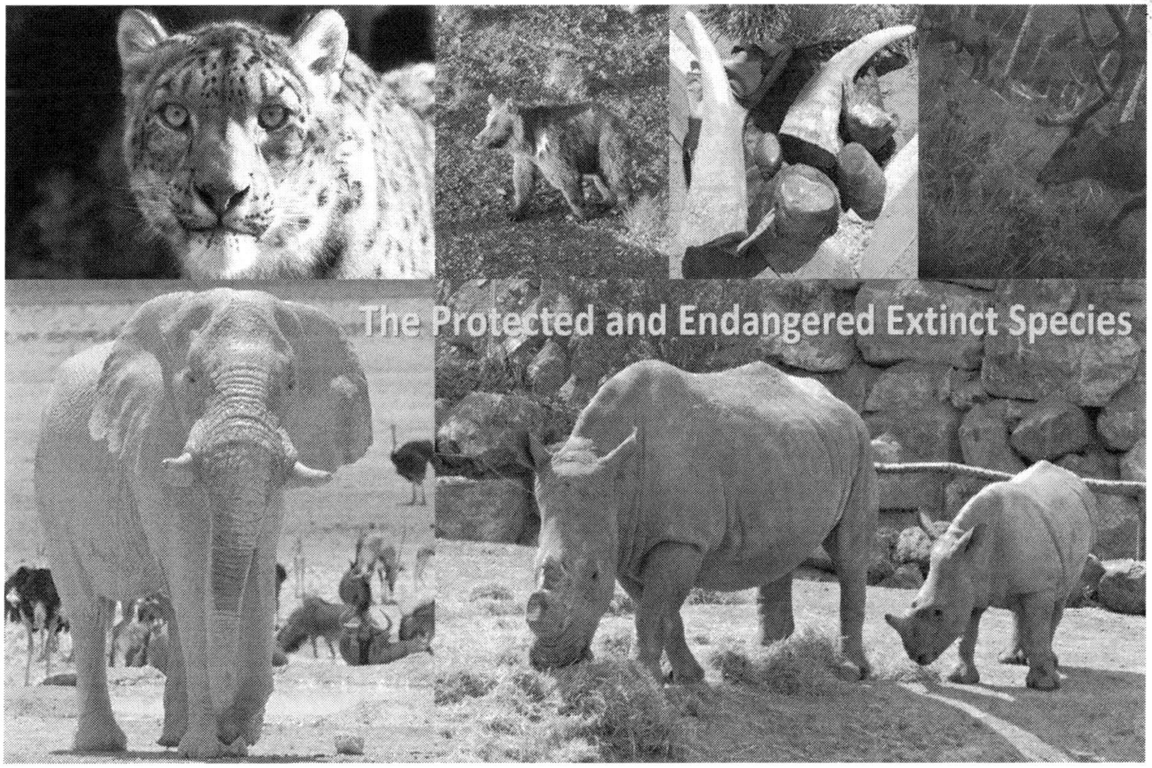

MICROORGANISM FACTS FOR KIDS

The Emergence of the Coronavirus

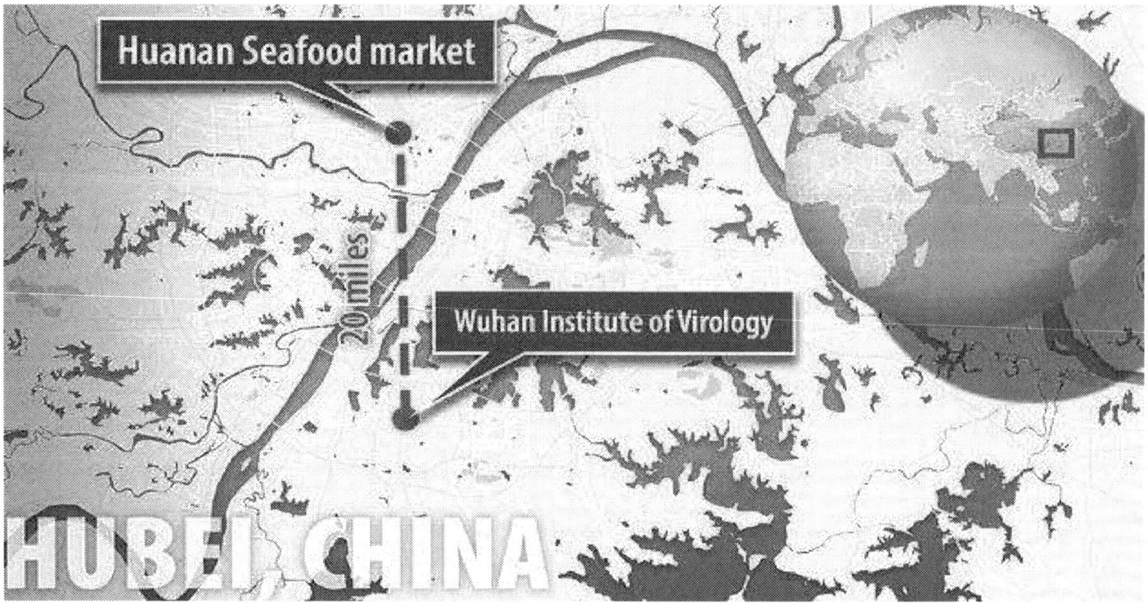

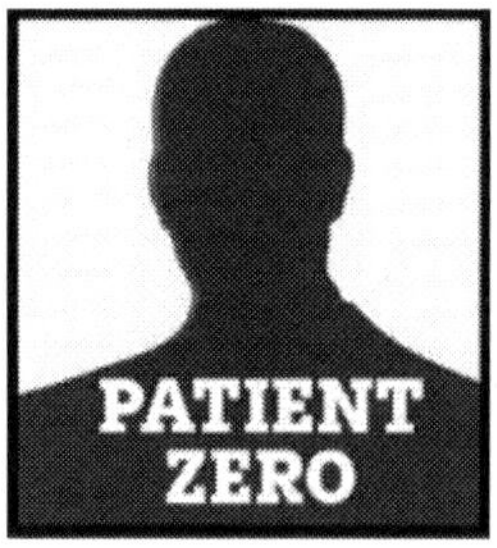

The novel coronavirus (2019-nCoV) disease emerged from an infected patient zero who resided in China Wuhan in December 2019. He was considered the first registered patient that had contracted the disease from an animal at a wet market based on the report released by the World Health Organisation.

To date, the exact origin of how the novel coronavirus comes about is still a mystery as virologists, genome and infectious disease experts can only establish findings based on genome analytical patterns extracted from millions of infected patients to give an assumption that the cause of the causative agent could probably derive from a contagious virus strains originated from wildlife animals such as bats, pangolins or even snakes that jumps into human transmission routes.

Some are still doubtful about its cause and made speculation that the whole propaganda can be a man-made biological warfare where one makes use of biological agents similar to the war archival in WWI and WWII's war history to carry out their mission of destruction in order to gain supremacy power control.

Trade-related sectors are being weighed down by a severe decline in external demand and supply chain disruptions except pharmaceutical manufacturing companies saw a spike demand for ventilators, masks and test kits requirements in this national crisis.

China Exotic Wildlife Market

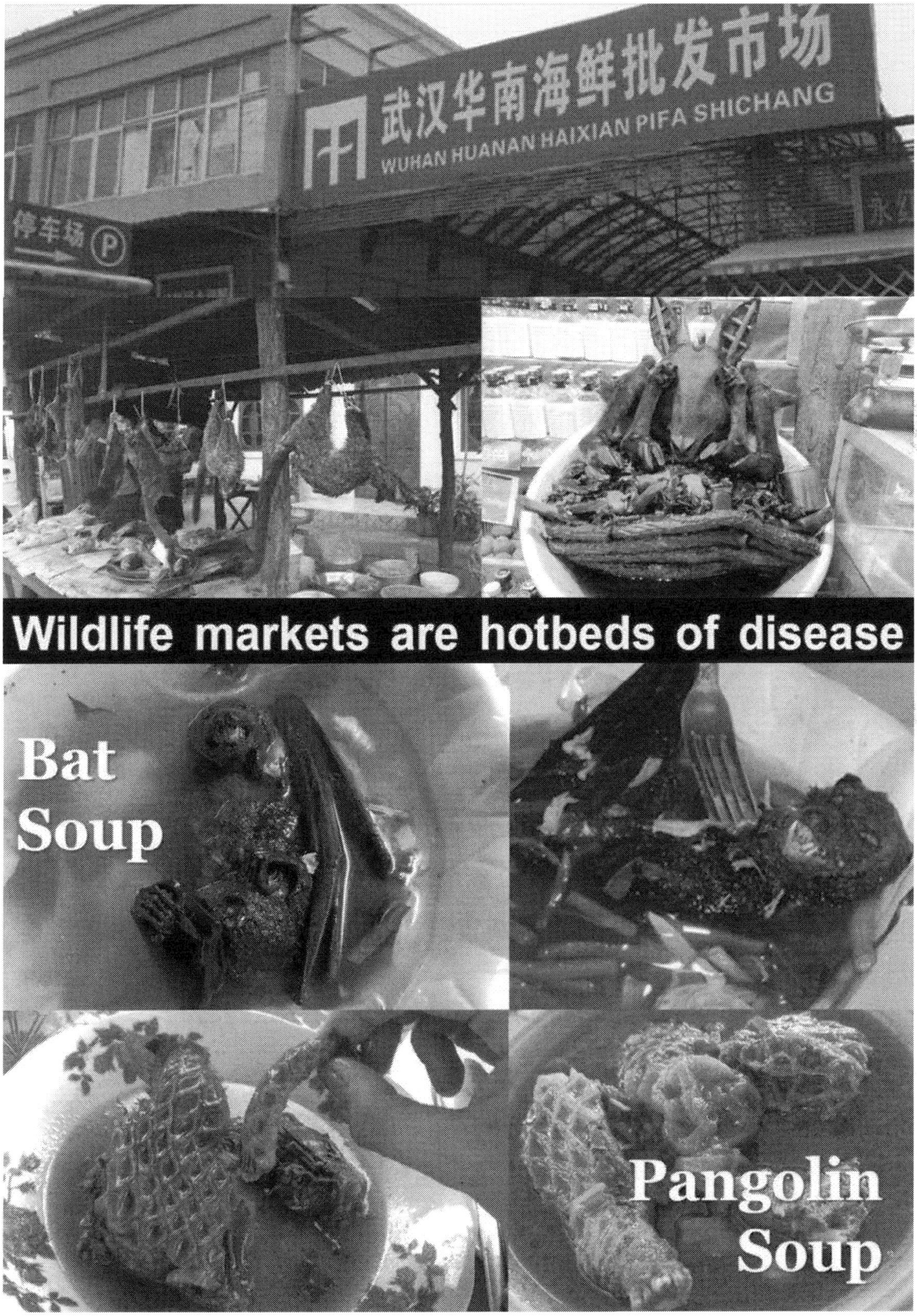

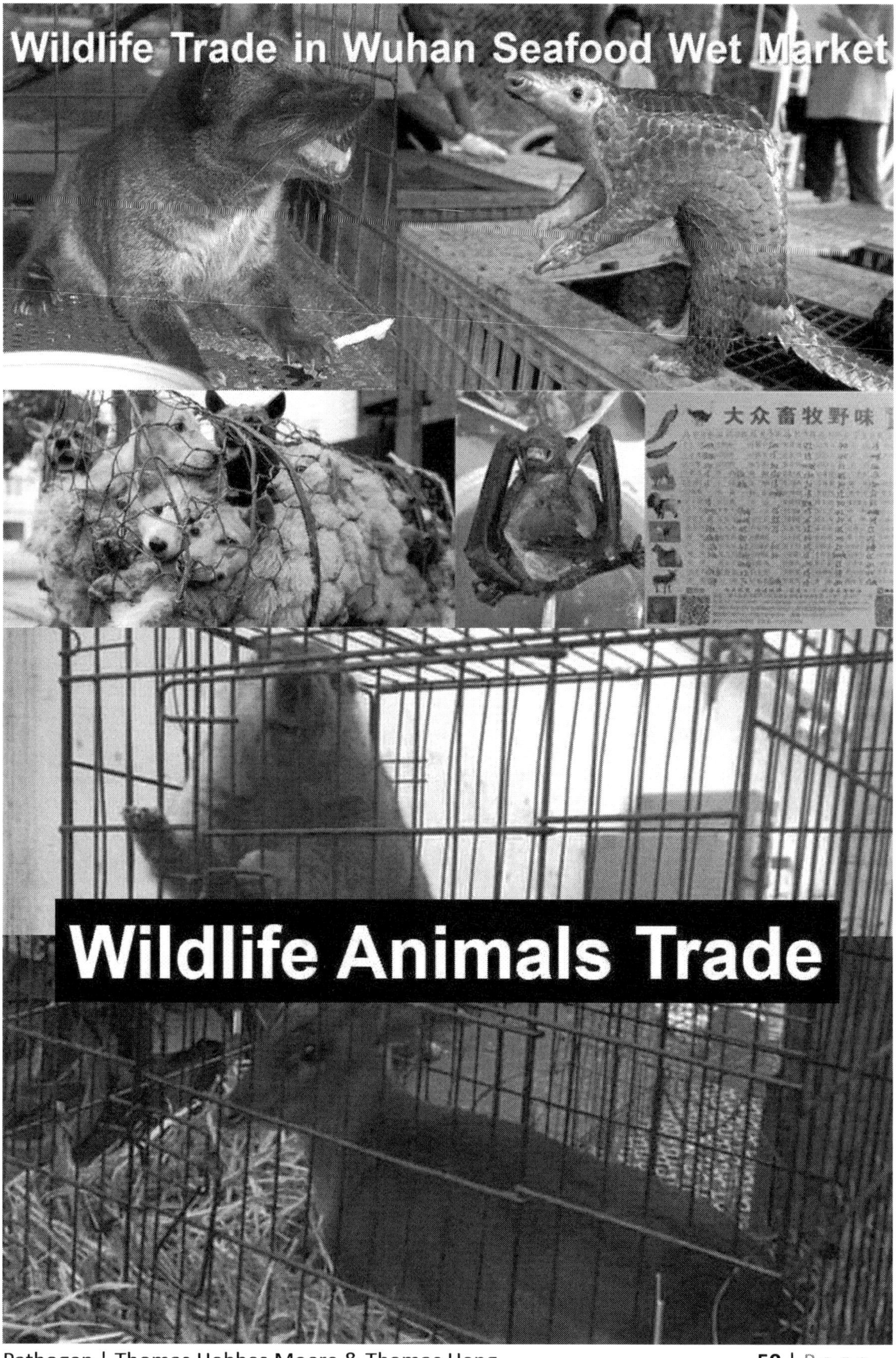
Wildlife Trade in Wuhan Seafood Wet Market
大众畜牧野味
Wildlife Animals Trade

Selling Animal Skins for Ornament Decorations

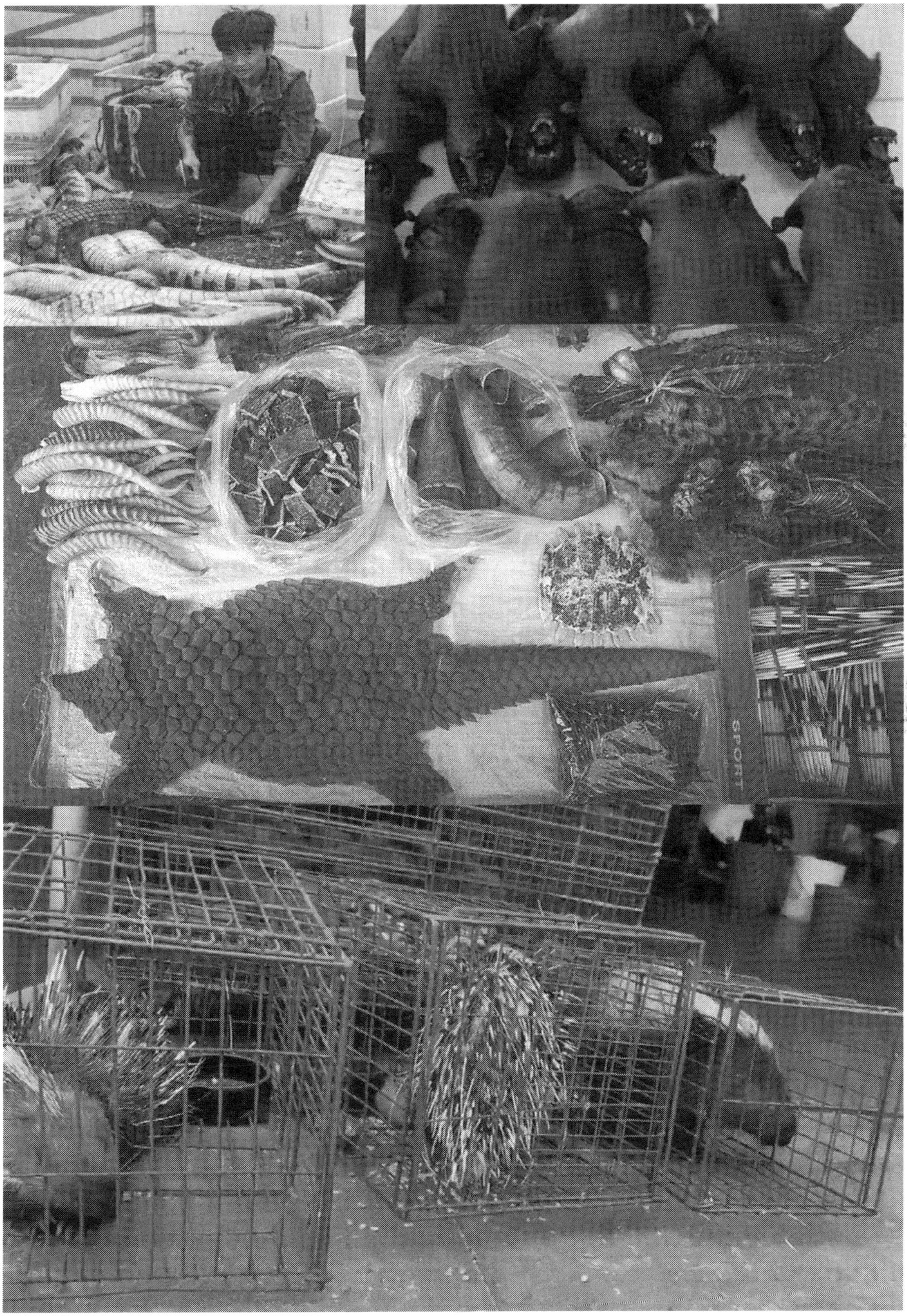

Selling Animals for Food Delicacy

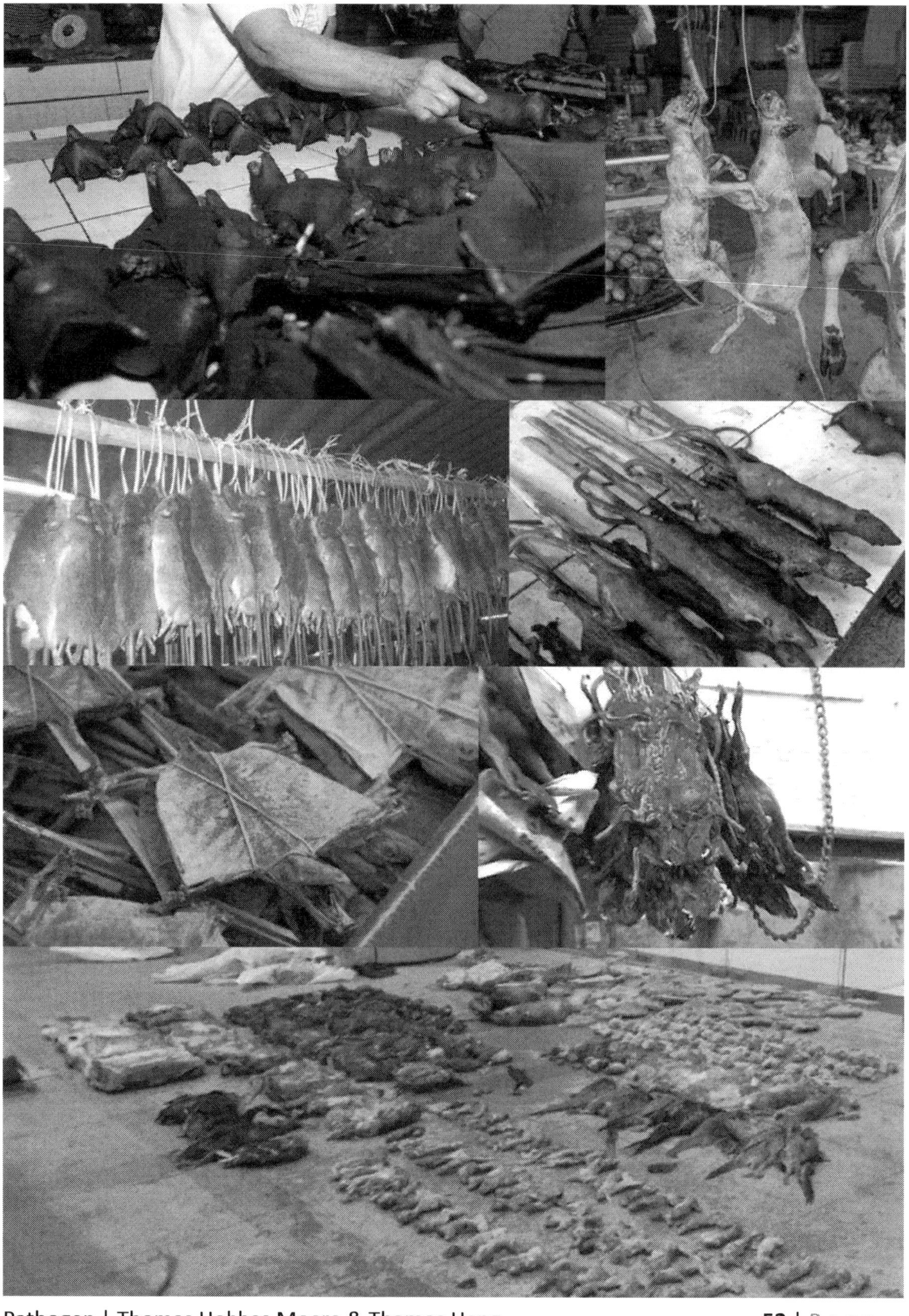

Microorganism Facts For Kids

Historical Toxic Gases and Biological Warfare

According to historical war archives, it reveals some fearful cases that ever happened using the most deadly man-made deployment of supertoxic gas or chemical warfare during WWI and germ warfare in WWII employing various methods in using infectious pathogen agents to incapacitate humans to gain tactical advantage over their enemies.

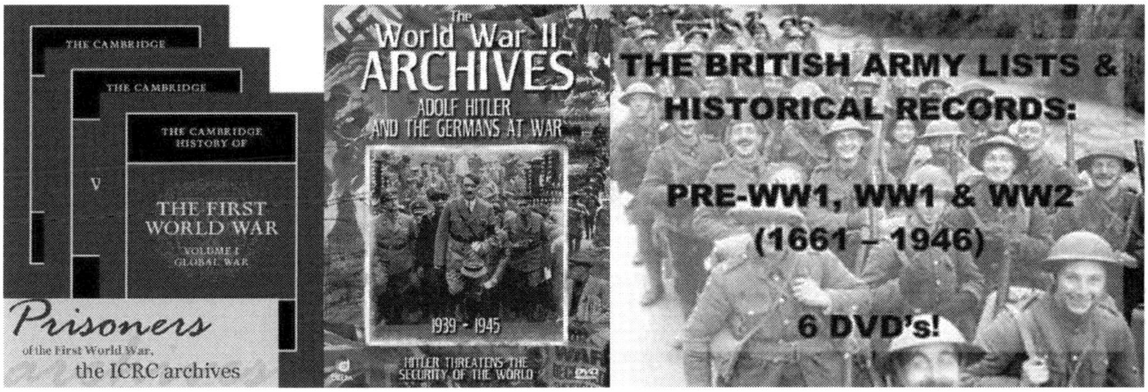

THE CAMBRIDGE
THE CAMBRIDGE
THE CAMBRIDGE HISTORY OF
THE FIRST WORLD WAR
VOLUME I GLOBAL WAR
Prisoners of the First World War, the ICRC archives
The World War II ARCHIVES
ADOLF HITLER AND THE GERMANS AT WAR
1939 - 1945
HITLER THREATENS THE SECURITY OF THE WORLD
THE BRITISH ARMY LISTS & HISTORICAL RECORDS:
PRE-WW1, WW1 & WW2
(1661 – 1946)
6 DVD's!

A Piece of A Past War History

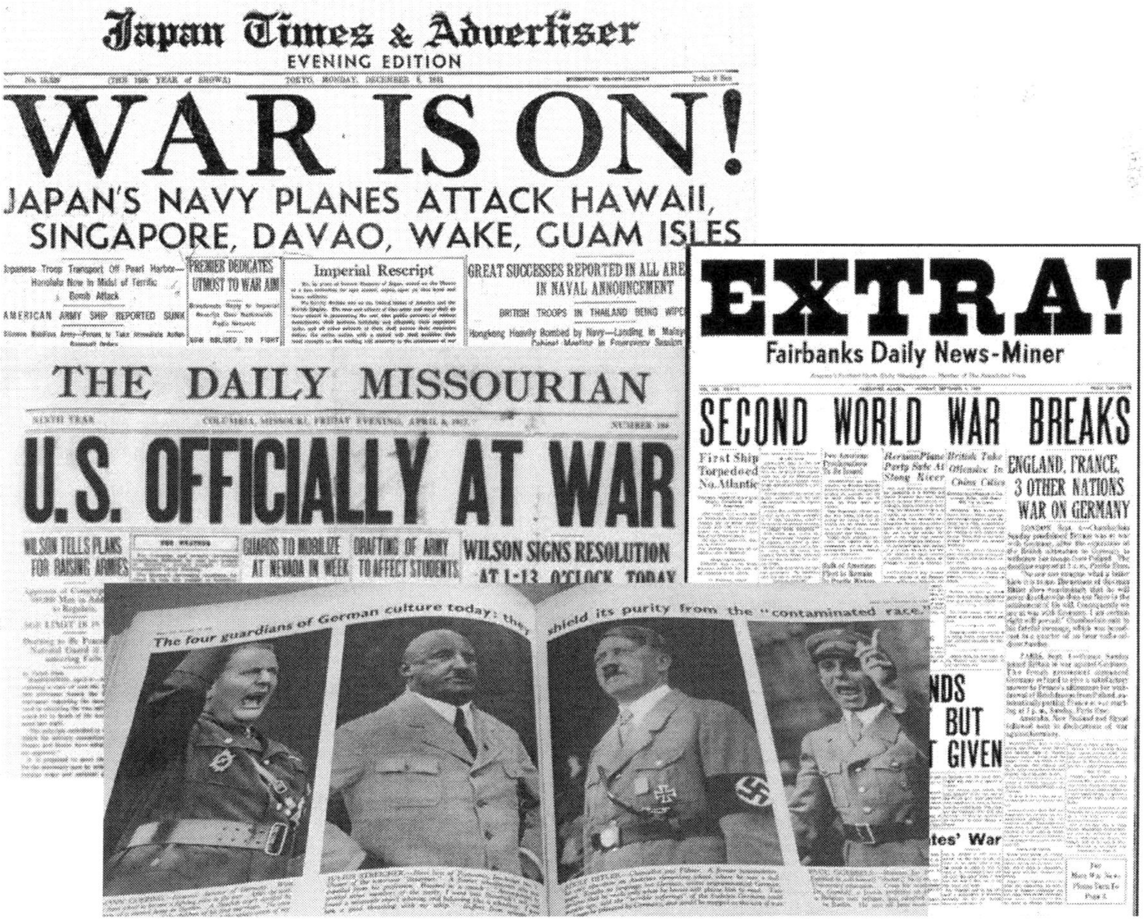

Japan Times & Advertiser
EVENING EDITION
WAR IS ON!
JAPAN'S NAVY PLANES ATTACK HAWAII, SINGAPORE, DAVAO, WAKE, GUAM ISLES
Imperial Rescript
GREAT SUCCESSES REPORTED IN ALL AREAS IN NAVAL ANNOUNCEMENT
EXTRA!
Fairbanks Daily News-Miner
SECOND WORLD WAR BREAKS
ENGLAND, FRANCE, 3 OTHER NATIONS WAR ON GERMANY
THE DAILY MISSOURIAN
U.S. OFFICIALLY AT WAR
WILSON SIGNS RESOLUTION
The four guardians of German culture today: they shield its purity from the "contaminated race."

During WWI war times, German Army used toxic chemicals and germs warfare to win the war by releasing toxic tear gas agents like phosgene, chlorine and mustard toxin gas to attack on their enemy base. Anthrax viruses were intentionally released to demoralize, injure and wipe up the whole enemy forces through the anthrax epidemic outbreak. Those infected were either dead or had to subject themselves to lifelong sufferings and pains in severe medical conditions beyond cure.

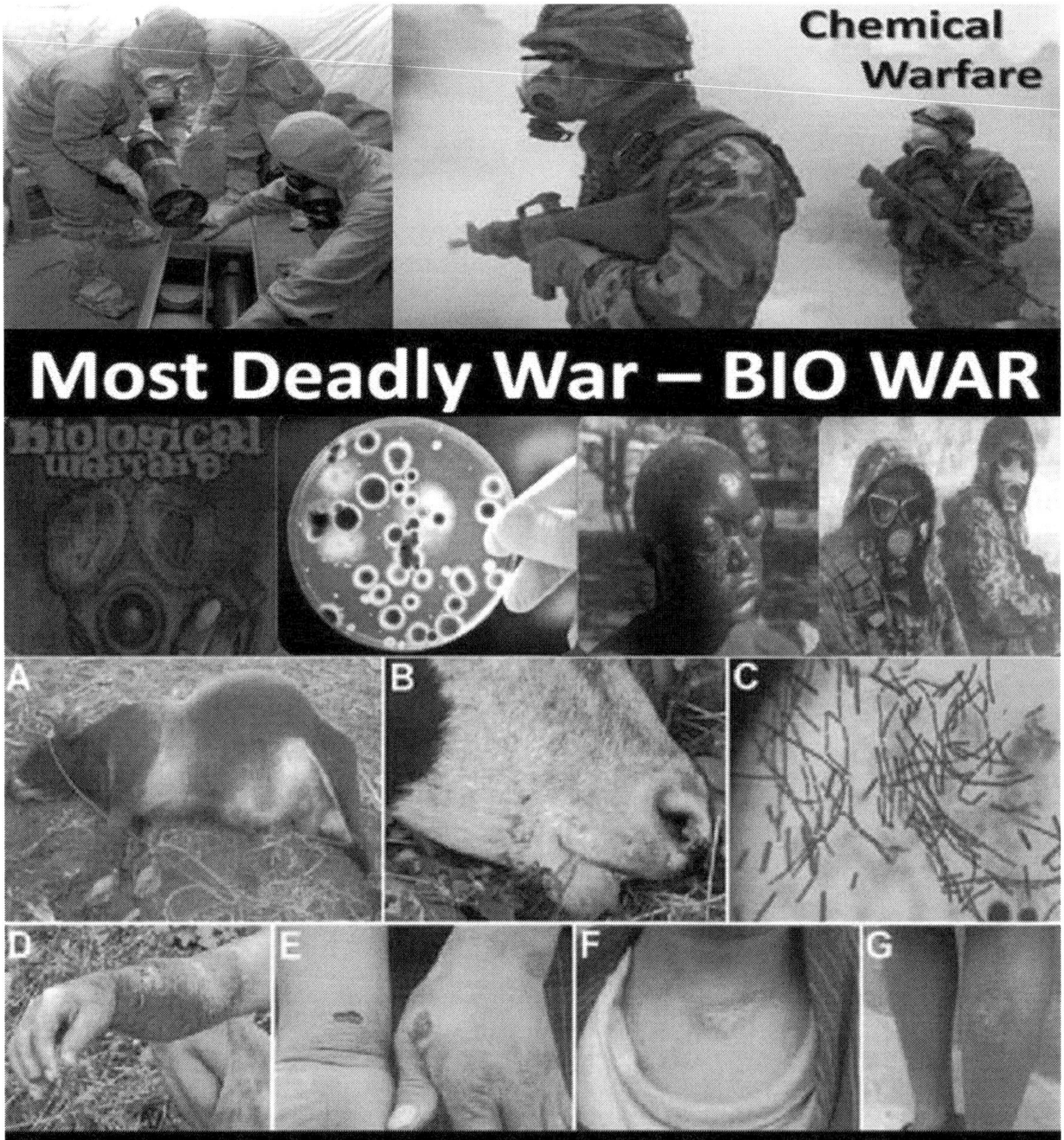

Signs of anthrax in infected animals (A–C) and humans (D–G), Bhutan, 2010. A) The carcass of an affected bull, showing bloating. B) Bleeding of unclotted blood from a cow's nostril. C) Rod-shaped Bacillus anthracis bacilli from 1 of the infected animals. Cutaneous anthrax causing severe inflammation of the arm (D) and typical black eschars on the hand and wrist (E), neck (scar) (E), and leg (G) of persons who had contact with B. anthracis –infected animals and carcasses.

MICROORGANISM FACTS FOR KIDS

Before World War II started, the Imperial Japanese Army had already been inspired by the German method of using lethal gas to attack on its ally's troops and wanted to apply the similar method to carry out the world invasion's conqueror ambitions. They then secretly sought their Japanese scientists to carry out an extensive research on it and commanded them to develop a lethal biological weapons for their strategic and tactical planning use in the coming war to gain supreme control power over the whole world.

For a decade, the Japanese scientists had been secretly involving a terrible human experimentation on their prisoners.

By using deadly pathogens to inject into their body with fatal and contagious organisms, many were made to suffer under the torturing of the diseases on cholera, anthrax, smallpox, and many other kinds of venereal diseases etc. and left them untreated in order to study and learn their side effects of the disease.

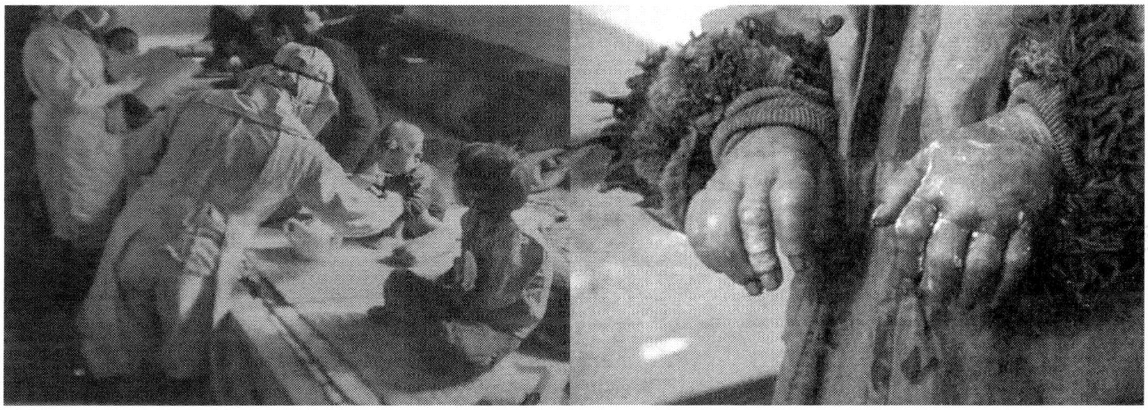

It is a horrific act and sufferings of humanitarian to the extreme that until today the older generation of the Chinese people had still not forgotten the miseries that they were forcibly made to undergo through the experimentation during the Japanese Occupation period.

The human pathogen experimentation was finally succeeded and the scientists were all getting ready to test and deploy a large-scale of biological weapons for the Imperial Japanese Army to use it on their war ambitions.

This episode led to World War II event when Unit 731 was formed to lead the whole Imperial Japanese Army to carry out their attack on China by using the lethal biological weapons that they had successfully tested and developed.

Microorganism Facts For Kids

Germs warfare attack were carried out in following manner of:

1. Planting bombs with deadly pathogens to extend its means of spread,
2. Water reservoirs and wells were secretly infected,
3. Aircrafts flew around the sky intentionally dropped tons of deadly bombs coupled with deadly pathogens into enemy territories but away from the Japanese army camps to infect allies' foods and clothing,
4. Plague-infected fleas were intentionally released to attack on the China army forces.

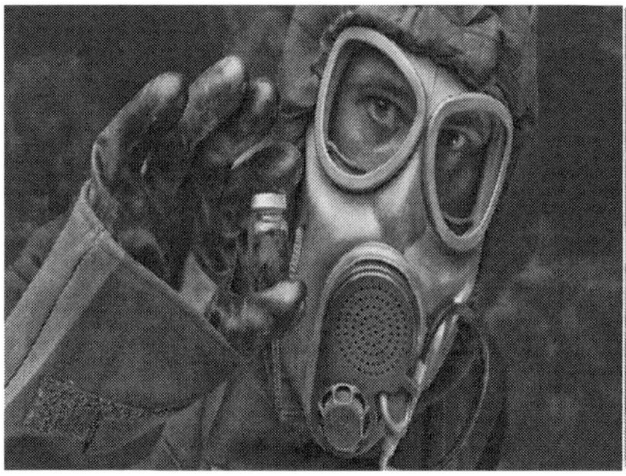
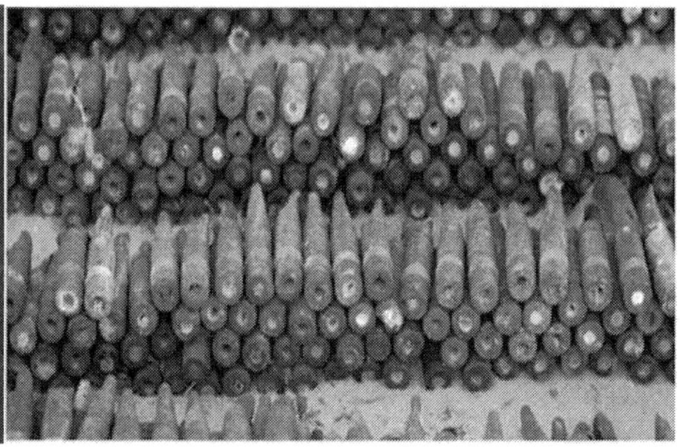

Unfortunately due to the unexpected change of wind and climate conditions, the uncontrollable spreading of the lethal pathogen agents had reversely affected many people, including the Japanese army troops who also became the victims of the deadly virus attacks.

Some of them died from the fatal diseases while other sufferers ended up with rotten legs and could no longer function their normal lives' activities ever again. Due to the terrible sufferings of many innocent victims after the warfare attacks, the deployment for both chemical and biological agent's warfare weapons are now prohibited and is considered a war crime tabled under a new constitution law.

The Biological Weapons Convention (BWC) came into force on March 26, 1975, leading to several disarmament international treaties being drawn up on April 10, 1972 for every states' leaders in the world to sign and agree upon for the mass destruction on their lethal agents to be disarmed, banning their invention, production and stockpiling supplies of biological weapons too. Any country engaged in the chemical and germ agents are now considered a war crime under the BWC treaties signed and attended by all States Party Leaders in the world.

BWC treaties signed and attended by all States Party Leaders in the world on April 10, 1972. It came into force on March 26, 1975

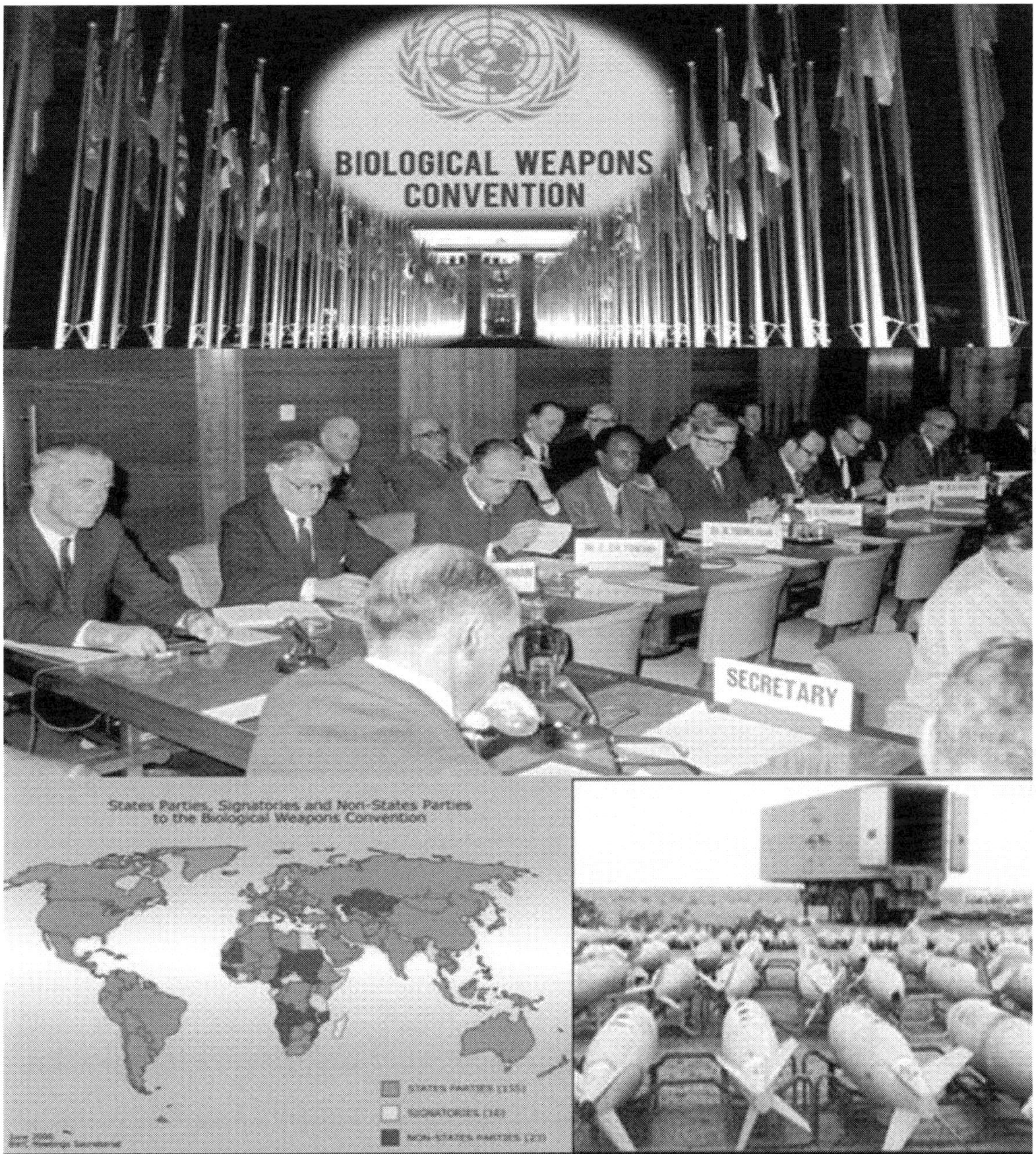

Banning Biological Weapons

- Geneva Protocol
  - ➢ Use of biological weapons was banned in international law by the Geneva Protocol of 1925
- Biological and Toxin Weapons Convention
  - ➢ The 1972 Biological and Toxin Weapons Convention extended the ban to almost all production, storage and transport of any types of biological weapons.

MICROORGANISM FACTS FOR KIDS

The Virus Infections Spread

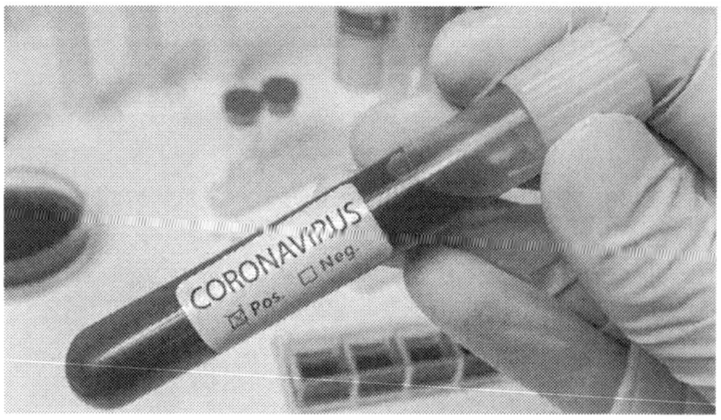

During the initial outbreak, the Chinese government was optimistic that they could contain this new virus, COVID-19, by quarantine the whole city of Wuhan and other nearby cities with a circumference area which covered about 50 million people inside Hubei province. But, unexpectedly it resulted in more alarming deaths coupled along with a spiral trend of uncontrollably confirmed and suspected infection cases every single day.

The Chinese scientists, virologist and infectious experts rallied together to carry out an extensive investigations over all the factual, scientific and bio data collated from millions of infected patients to conclude the result that this disease was far capable to infect human transmissions. No vaccine is effective to treat this infections. Besides that, they also discover that those infected who had recovered mysteriously were mainly due to their strong immune functionality capable to fight the bug on its own.

Flash News and updates were broadcasted daily on alert warnings. Precautionary measures by advisory health authority were constantly flashed to advise public to wash hands frequently, wear mask and adopt social distancing as part of the health safety preventive measures.

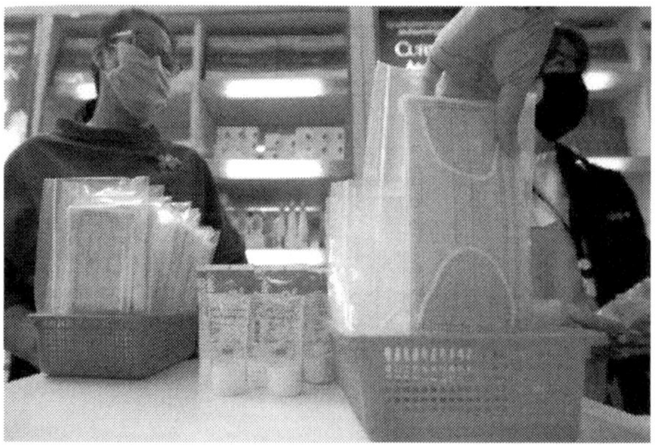

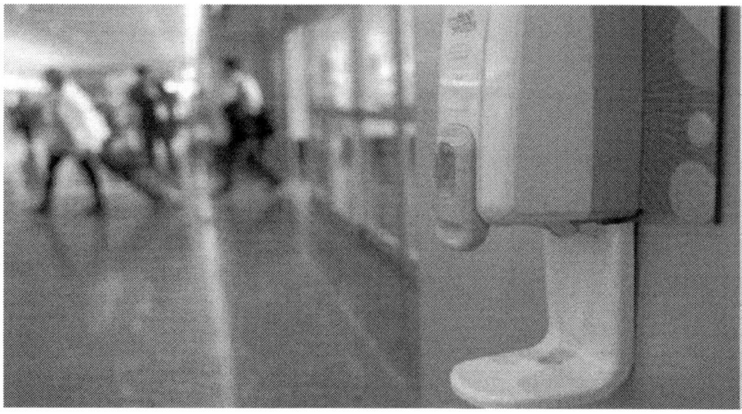

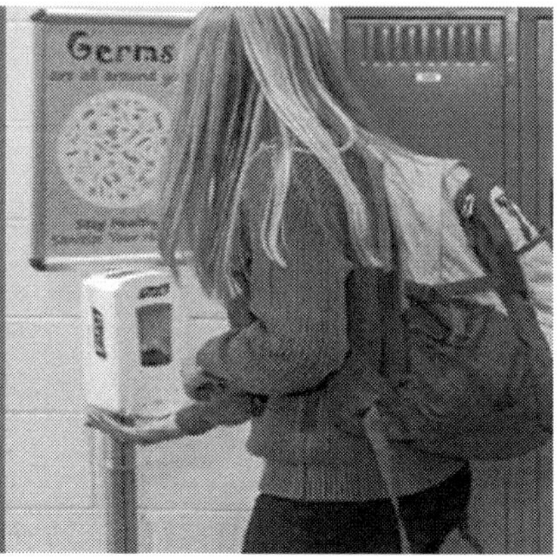

Surgical masks were issued to the public and hand sanitizer dispensers were visibly put up at all public essential service areas for daily use.

The Chinese government alerted WHO on 31 Dec 2019 on its severity impact. WHO then declared it raise a red flag to the world an international health emergency a "Pandemic" Coronavirus Outbreak on 30 January 2020. This new virus was given a name COVID-19 under the coronavirus family.

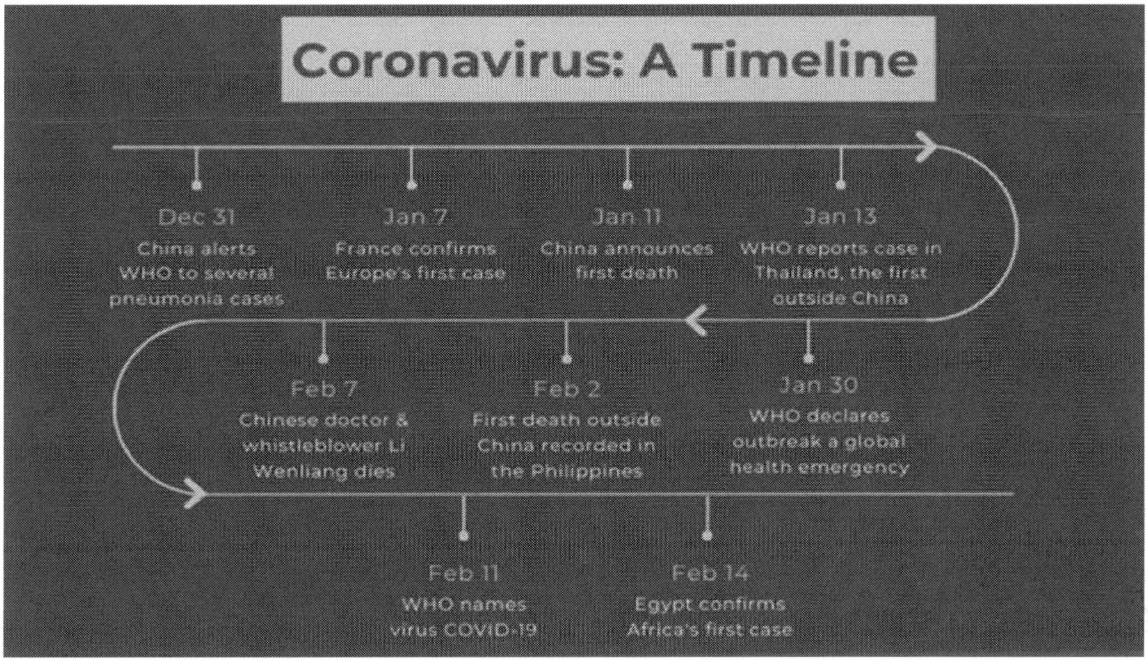

To date, the spread of this new virus infections had hampered the global trade and economic growth on the world economy and the battling of the pandemic situation is seen far worse than the Great Depression times.

During the Great Depression times, a global crisis that ever happened lasted for 10 years of severe economic depression from 1929 to the late 1939s that saw millions of investments being wiped out from the turmoil stock market. Many people had lost their job and businesses went under bankruptcy as a result. Suicidal, family woes, divorce cases were on the rise during this trying times which had the similar outcomes like today events.

In China, the Chinese government begins to implement lockdown for months to slow down the spread of the virus infection, shutting down airports, entertainment centers, eateries and even schools to the extent of banning funerals and weddings gathering on site and all other non-essential shops as well until the situation improves.

A legislative mandatory law was passed down swiftly, requiring every person to wear a face mask when out and about and no forming of group gatherings to be seen under any circumstances. Social gathering was disallowed.

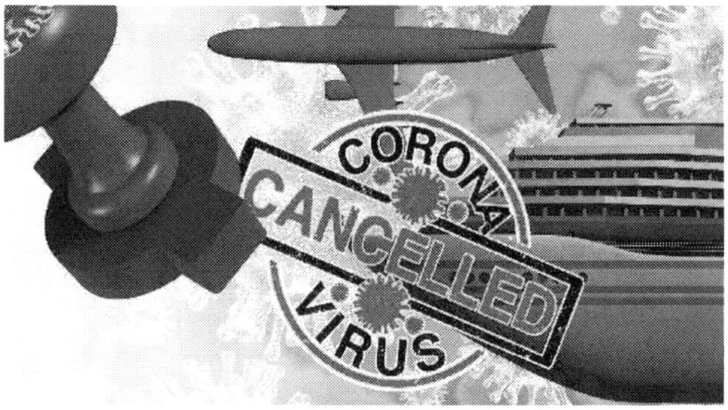

Under the Infectious Diseases Act, an enforcement officer could take stern action against violators if individuals, business owners or entities flouted the orders and requirements.

Officers and COVID-19 ambassadors were deployed to control the situation and ensuring that the public adhered to the protocols for their own health safety precautions.

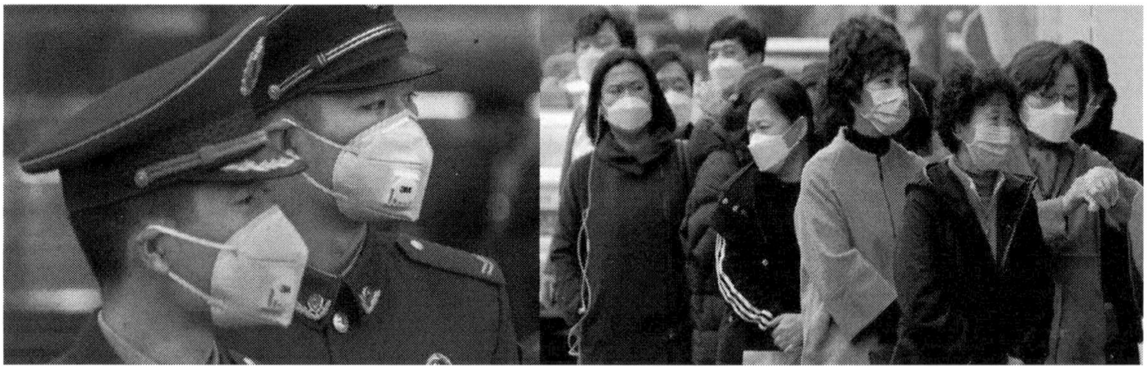

People were advised to stay indoors and used telecommuting technology to work from home. Even school children were not made exceptional. Children stay at home to use tele-video conferencing to interact with their school lessons from their relevant school teachers.

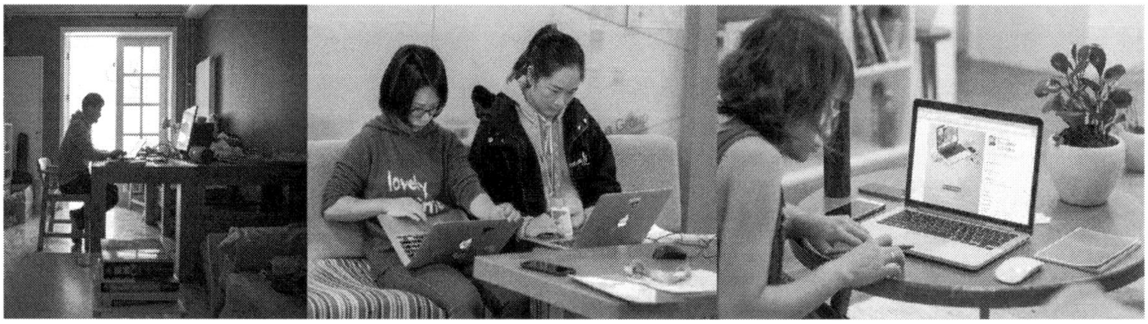

If the virus infection cases still remained uncontrollable, the lockdown period would be extended with more stringent measures to be imposed to curb the coronavirus transmission by further minimising human interaction.

MICROORGANISM FACTS FOR KIDS

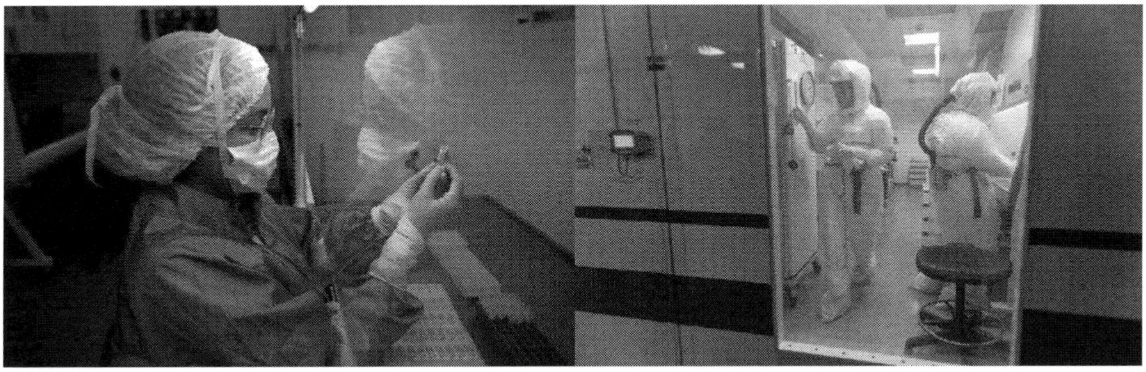

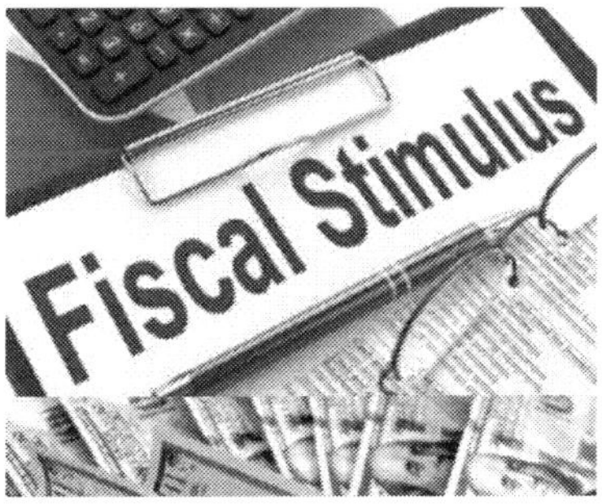

Economic challenges were an uphill fight. Every nation leader across the globe was rolling out stimulus financial relief packages to help cushioning the hardship their citizens are facing now and then to help them tide over this difficult times while fighting the bug together as one unified team spirit.

On the other hand, billions of dollars are also pumped in to find a vaccine for the coronavirus cure as scientists in the world are racing against time as the infection cases keep going up globally.

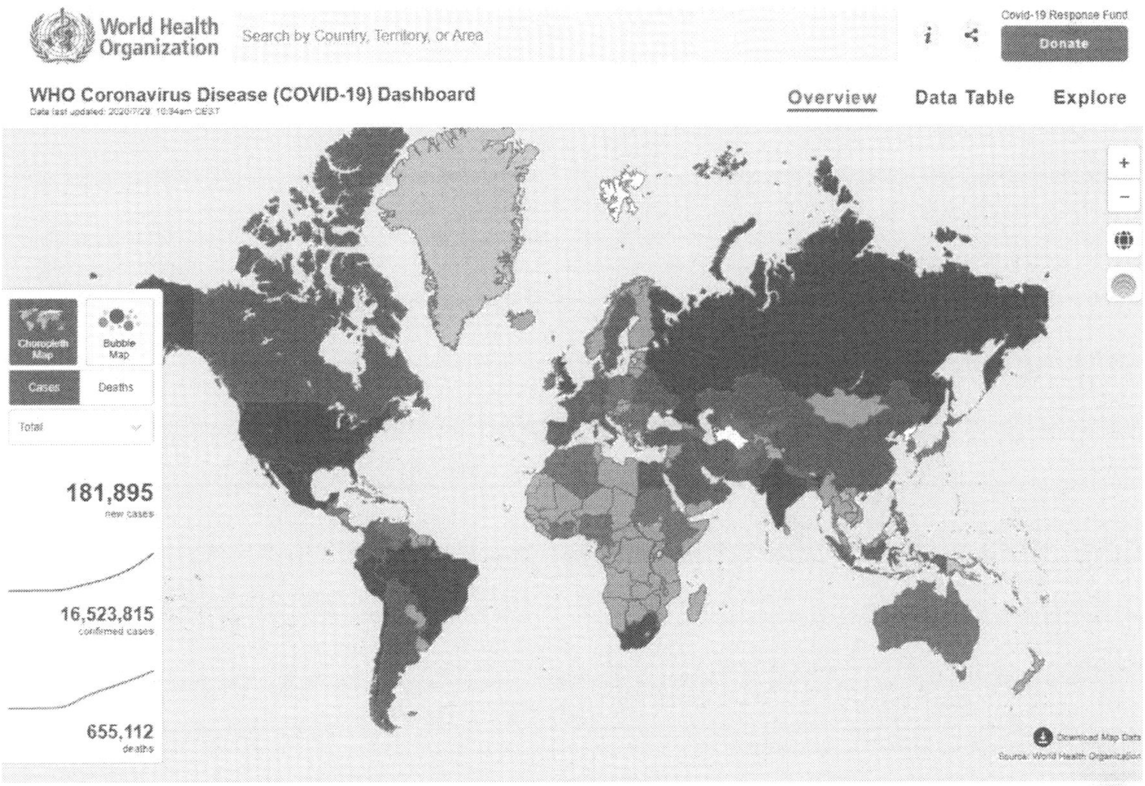

Globally, as of 10:34am CEST, 29 July 2020, there have been 16,523,815 confirmed cases of COVID-19, including 655,112 deaths, reported to WHO.

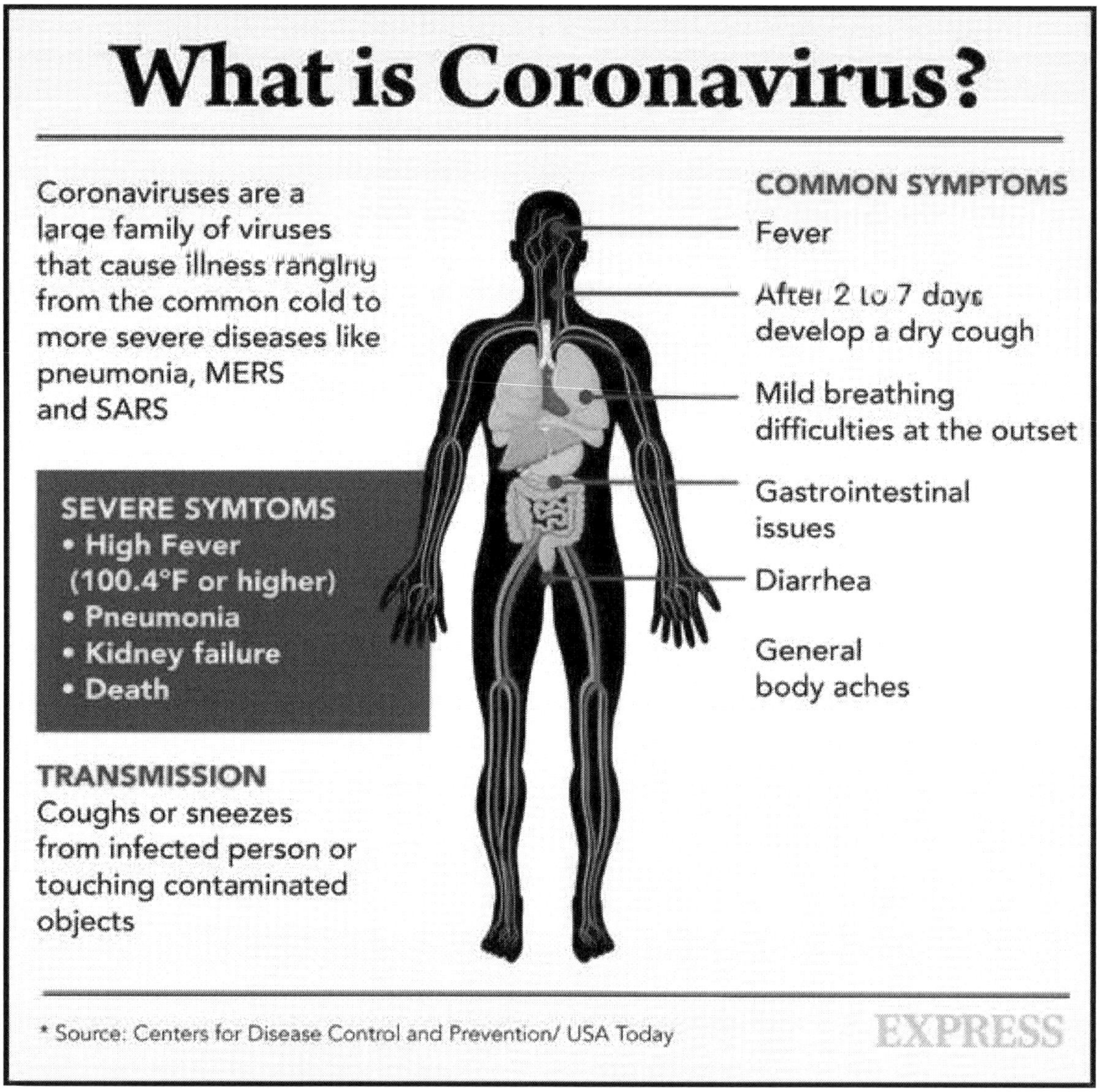

Corona means “crown” in Latin and the virus appears like wearing a spiky crown under a microscopic.

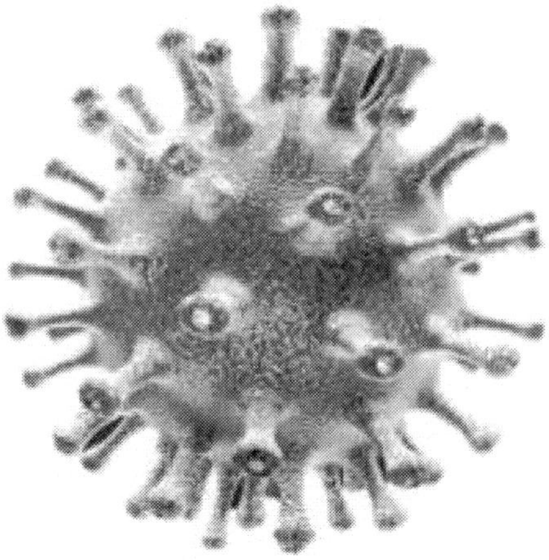

Until today, nobody including medical experts knows for sure what and where this mystery animal come from that cross jumps from another type of animal and transmits the germ to humans. But some people believe it can be the pangolin, a scaly animal that eats ants instead of bat which originally was thought to be the case. And some even say that it is actually come from snake.

MICROORGANISM FACTS FOR KIDS

How Coronavirus Makes People Sick

Coronavirus is an influenza which comes under the family umbrellas of SARS, Severe Acute Respiratory Syndrome. It mainly affects the lung regions through mostly in droplets form.

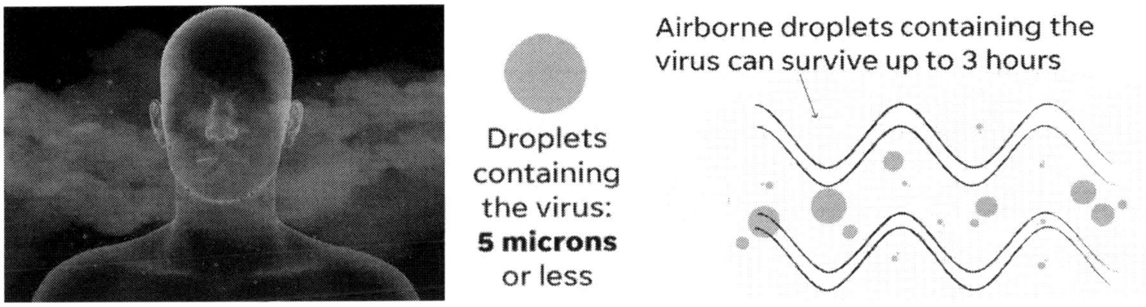

Coronavirus signs and symptoms usually show up with:

1. Fever
2. Dry cough
3. Running nose
4. Loss of Taste Bug and Smell
5. Breathing difficulties

People exhibit such symptoms are suggested to stay away from crowds and to impose self-quarantine for 14 days isolation at home. They have to keep tab on their own temperature by monitoring twice a day to ensure themselves are not positive COVID-19.

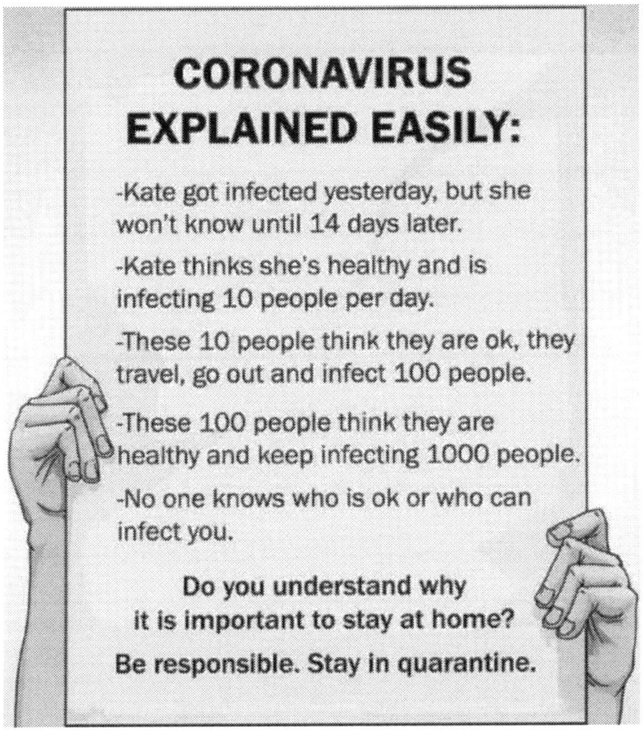

During the 14 days isolation period, if there is no fever symptom showing up at all until the last day, they can then leave their home and resume for work and their normal daily activities.

If any of the above symptom shows up, they need to immediately see doctor for follow up actions.

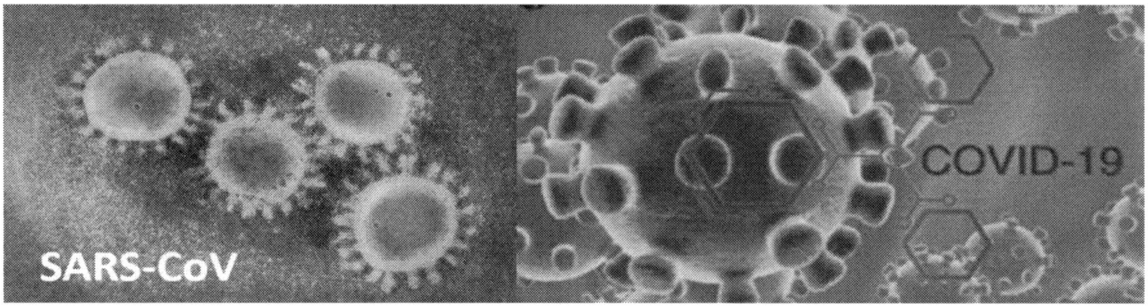

After detailed studies carry out on the new virus patterns, COVID-19 and other SARs viruses, they found similarity among them with a crown-like patterns. COVID-19 as a result is concluded.

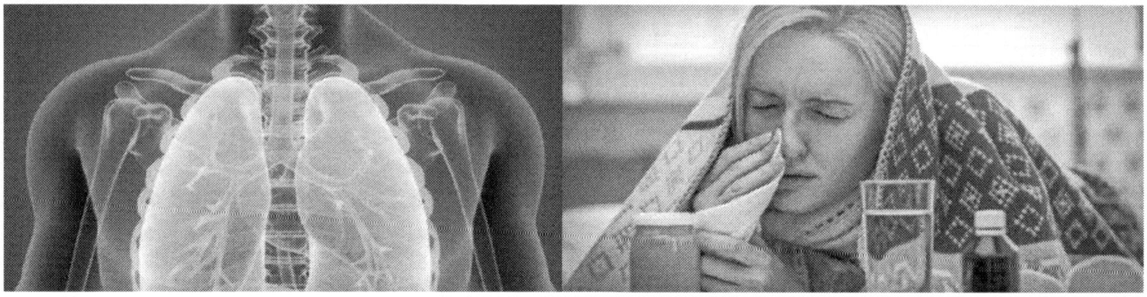

They can spread by droplets transmission through the air. Infected person when coughing, sneezing, from saliva droplets or nose mucous can discharge the germs into the air or leave behind contaminated tiny particles onto any surfaces that they come in contact with.

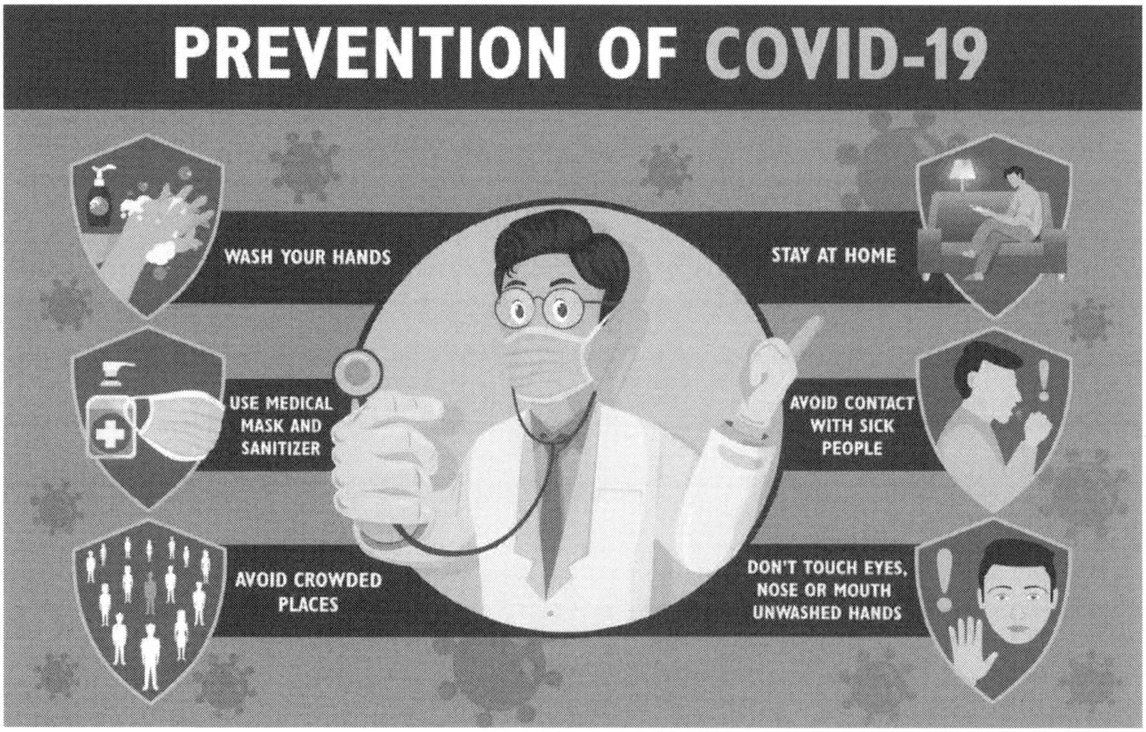

The Coronavirus Timeline Infections

The novel coronavirus, SARS-CoV-2, travels from the upper respiratory pathway from the throat to the lungs region and finally on the veins' bloodstream, taking from Wuhan's 200 patients disease timeline progression being published in Lancet medical journal.

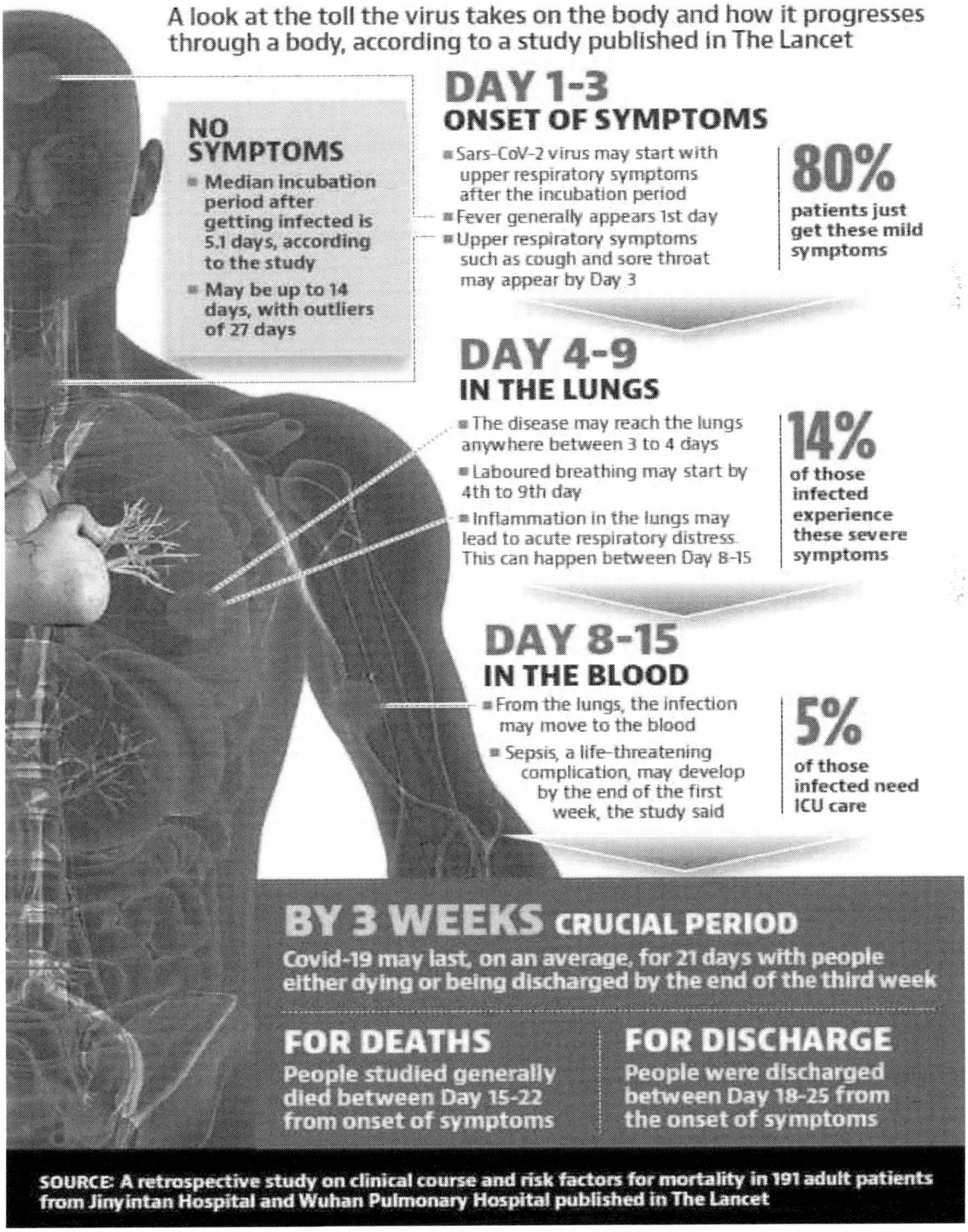

Don't Underestimate the Coronavirus Attack

Do not overlook the liver as there are real cases that happened to novel coronavirus patients.

Case#1 Damaged Liver

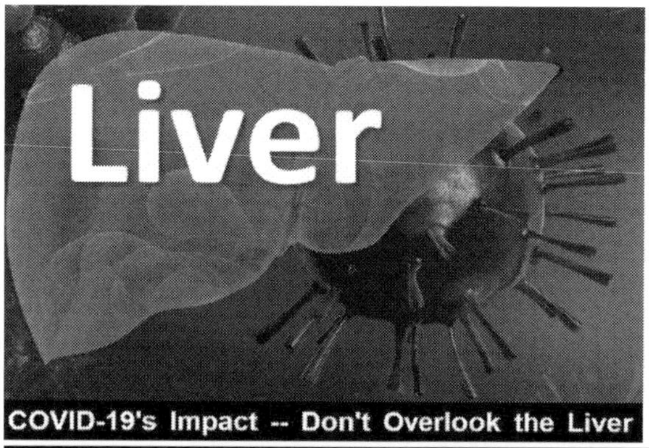

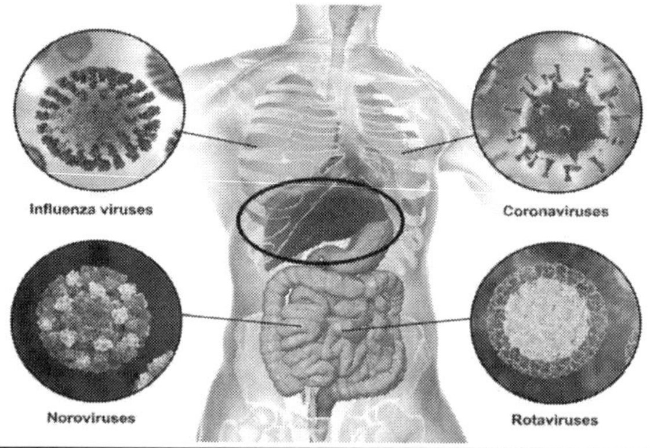

Wuhan doctors who were critically ill with coronavirus wake up to find that their skin has turned dark after virus damaged their liver

By Billie Thomson For Mailonline
18:31 20 Apr 2020, updated 19:38 20 Apr 2020

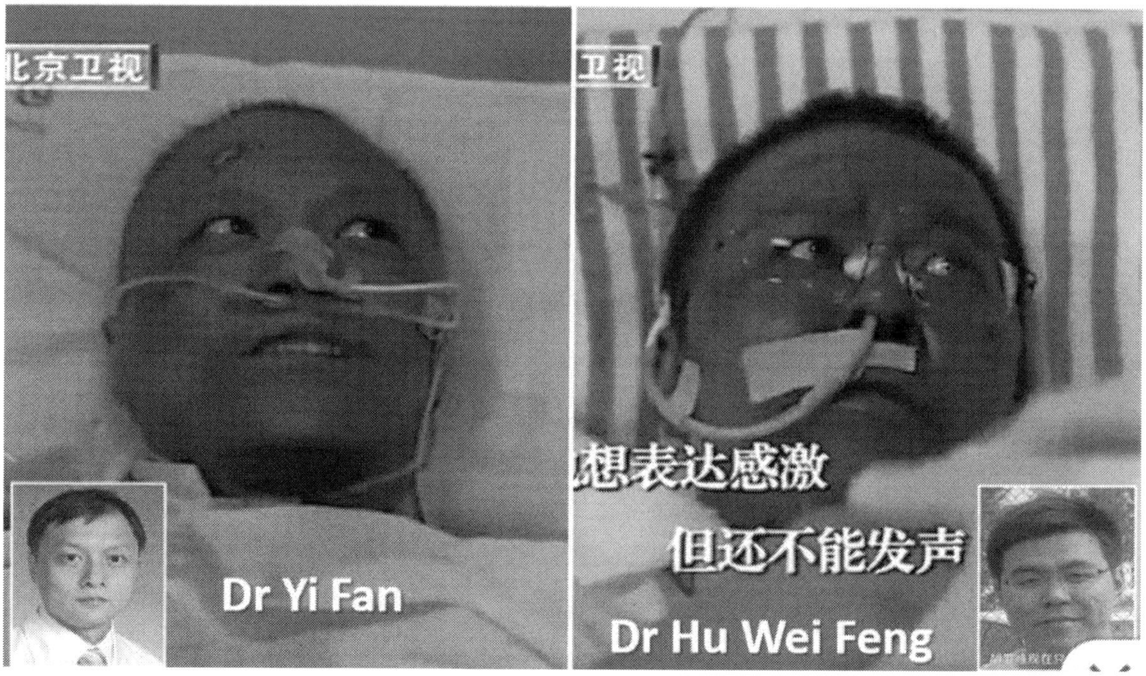

In January 2020, the Chinese doctors by the name of Dr Yi Fan, a cardiologist, and Dr Hu Wei Feng, a urologist, who were colleagues working at Wuhan Central Hospital with Dr Li Wen Liang, the whistle blower who died of the gravely infection on 7 February 2020, were also both diagnosed and tested positive COVID-19 while treating patients in the month of January.

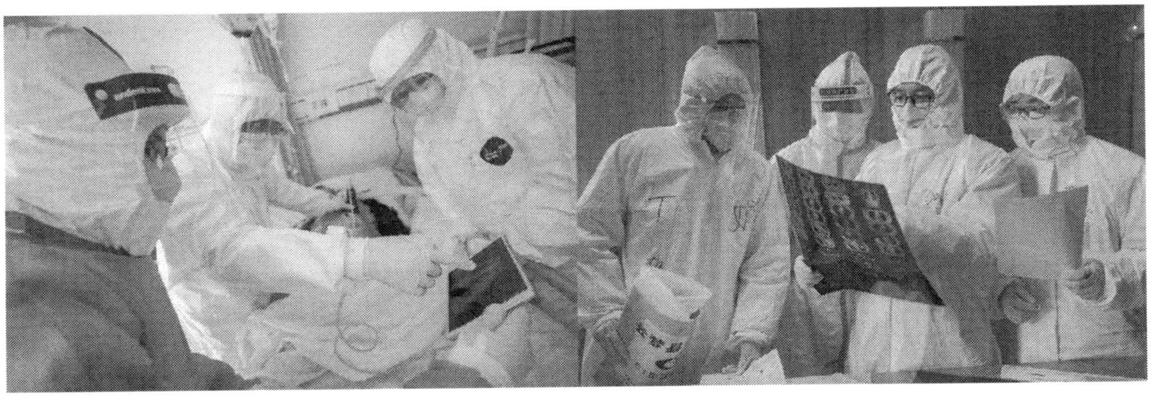

Both were bedridden ever since. After struggling for four months of intensive treatment at Wuhan Pulmonary Hospital, they finally woke up from their coma stage to find that their skin pigments had already turned to a darker tone as a result of the liver damage believed to be the cause of the deadly virus infections. Both men received a terrible shock in their life after they got to know their illness conditions.

Physically they felt immensely weak but mentally they went through a psychological traumatic experience in accepting the truth facts. Since then, their stories were published on every media and became well known as the two black-faced Wuhan doctors. Praises were kept pouring in for their bravery fighting spirit against the killer disease.

China Daily reported that Dr Yi Fan was only discharged on 6 May 2020. But, sadly, Dr Hu Wei Feng appeared never to recover from the ordeal and finally succumbed to his death on 2 June 2020 from the deadly disease complications after battling with it for nearly five months since January.

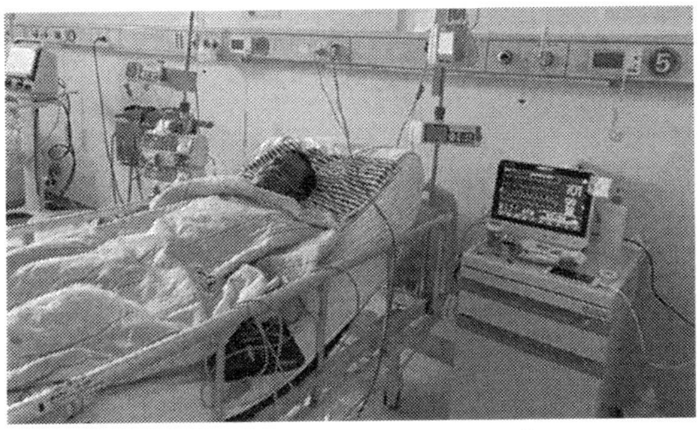

According to local state media reported on 2 June 2020, he had become the sixth doctor from the epicentre Wuhan to have died of the disease since the first COVID-19 fatality emerged in December 2019.

Case#2 Mysterious Blood Clots

Doctors are paying attention to the coronavirus disease discovery in a way that they have found blood clots in patients' lungs area.

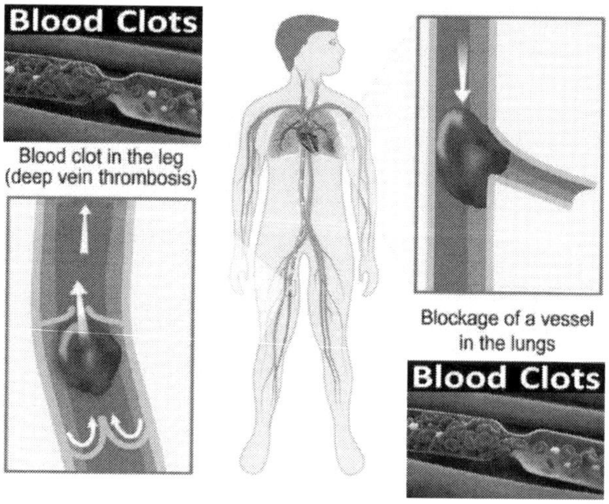

From the patient's X-rays taken, it shows that the lung areas are surrounded with hundreds of microclots that are causing acute respiratory distress syndrome known as "wet lung" to the sick patient.

Wet lung syndrome in patients is mainly caused by microclots which attribute to the lack of blood flow from the lungs during which the blood carries less oxygen leaving the lungs. This explains why ventilator operates poorly for patient with low blood oxygen as a result.

Microclots can lead patient to lethal pulmonary embolisms, strokes, heart attacks, kidneys and other chronic issues as well.

Risk Factors for Pulmonary Embolism (PE)

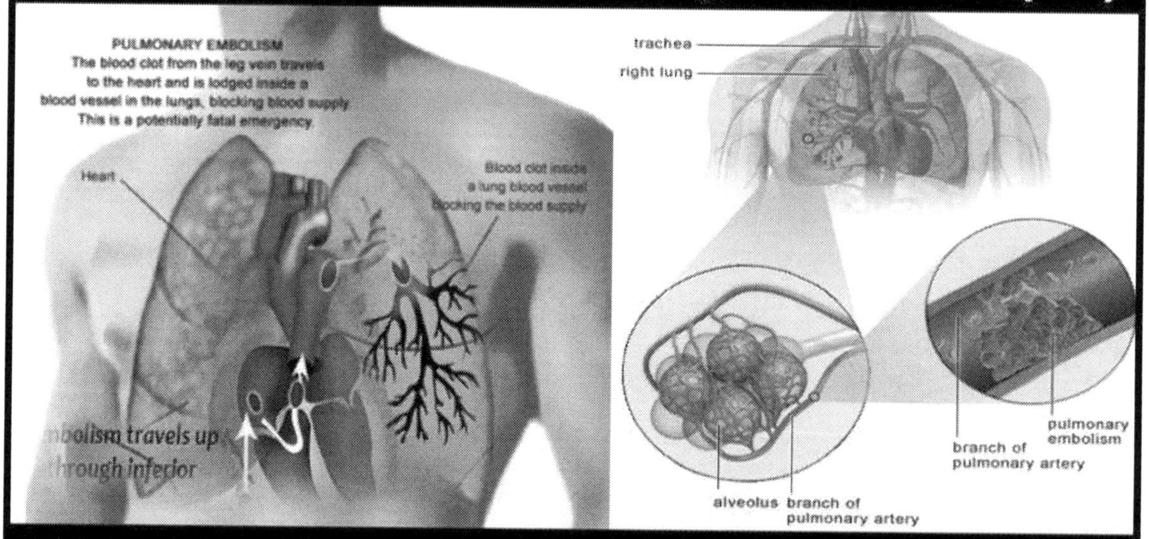

PE travels up through inferior vena cava to heart and lungs

The pulmonary embolus syndrome prevents the action of exchanging oxygen and carbon dioxide in the lungs and also restrict the amount of blood flow reaching to the lungs.

MICROORGANISM FACTS FOR KIDS

Patients with blood clots are usually critically ill and need to be admitted to the ICU wards for constant monitoring. Others will have severe complications like kidney issues and heart problems and need to be hooked up to a ventilator pumping machines to assist them with their breathing difficulties in their lungs.

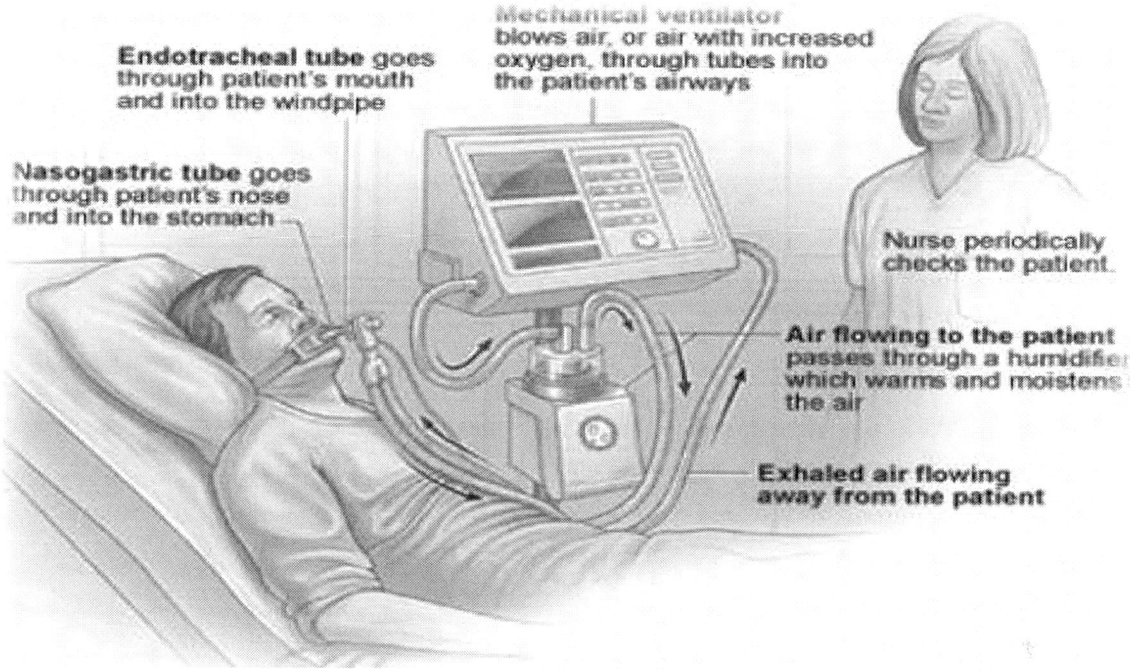

A patient with blood clot issues usually experience a severe intense limbs' pain over his entire body. This is because the person blood supply to the limb is blocked and the nourishment and oxygen cannot reach the nerve and muscle cells. As a result when he tries to bend over, lift up his hand, arm and leg or even stretch his little finger, he can feel very painful.

If there is really a severe lack of blood flow to both feet and hands, an amputation will be the last call for the doctor to carry out an emergency operation on the patient to save his life so that his other parts of the organs will not be severely damaged too.

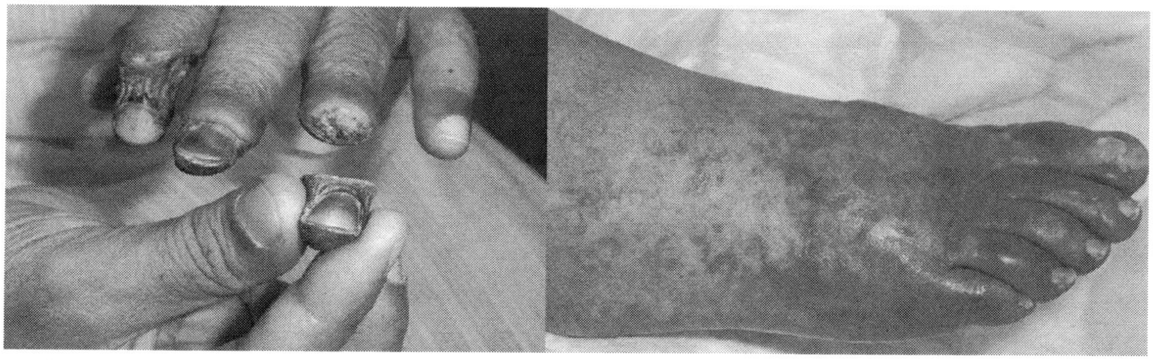

Case#3 Neurological Symptoms Lead to Paralysis Effects

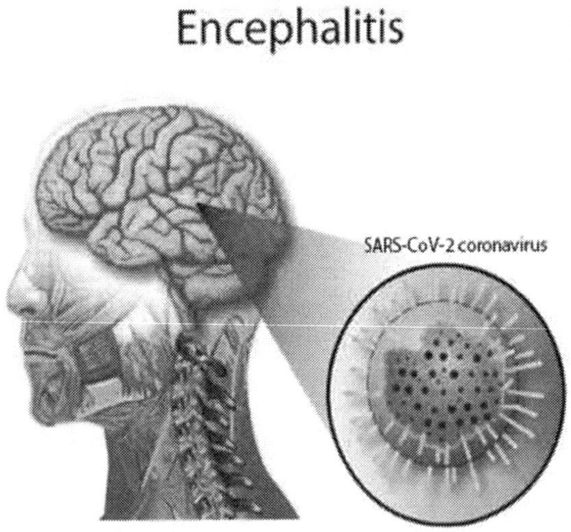

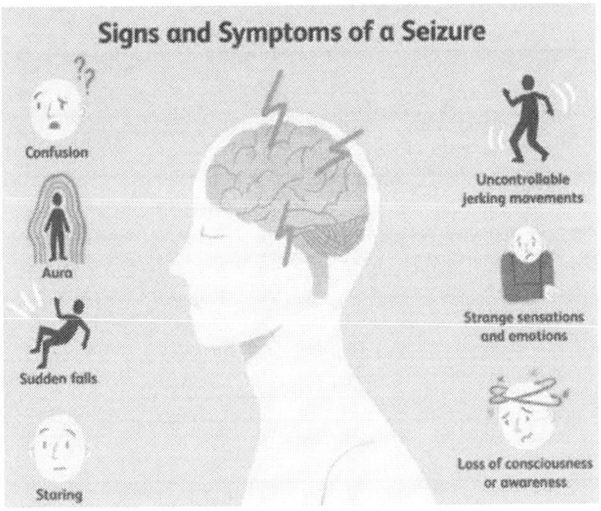

There are cases reported that coronavirus patient also experiences muscle weakness, viral encephalitis (inflammation of the brain) and seizures medical conditions. As a result, doctors are now worrying if patient suddenly develops neurological symptoms, he may become paralyse and the younger patient is not spared from the episode too.

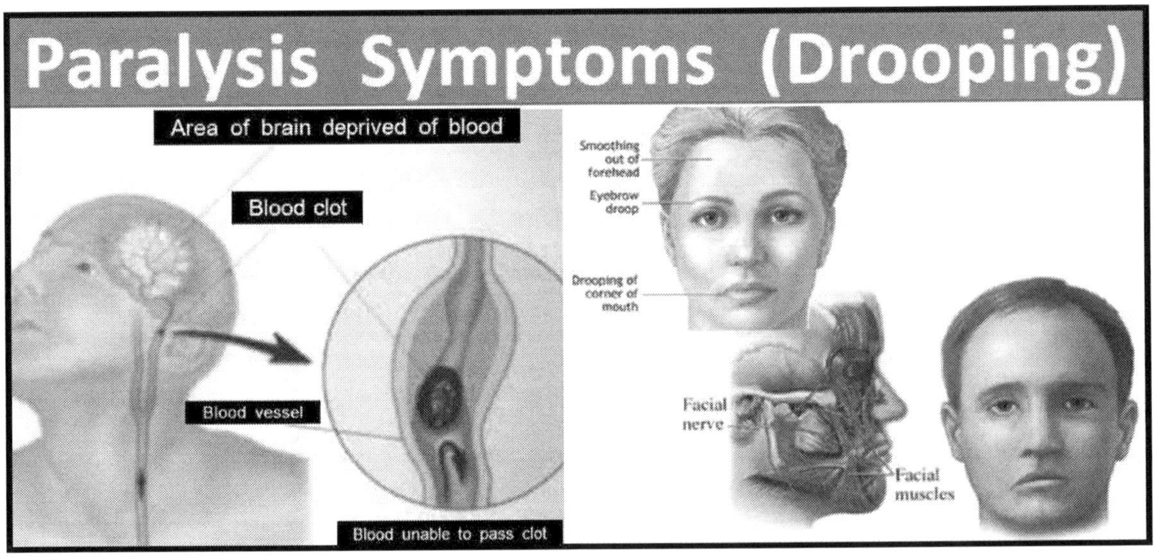

Based on the global scientific findings and studies on the coronavirus family, SARS-CoV-2 coronavirus disease cannot be underestimated its fatalities. It can severely cause damages to the central nervous system from the lungs, heart all the way to the brain.

The nervous system can cause illness symptoms such as headache, dizziness, disturbance of consciousness, acute cerebrovascular disease inclusive of epilepsy and peripheral neuropathy conditions.

Microorganism Facts For Kids

Peripheral neuropathy condition can create an intricate nerves network system. It carries messages to and fro from the brain as well as from the spinal cord all the way to the muscles, skin and internal organs.

Any impairment along the pathway can lead to peripheral neuropathy.

Patient as a result experiences sudden weakness, nerves sensitivities like numbness and pain all over his whole body, deteriorating taste and smell, and loss appetite. In general, besides respiratory symptoms, doctors also need to monitor closely to the manifestations of neurological symptoms.

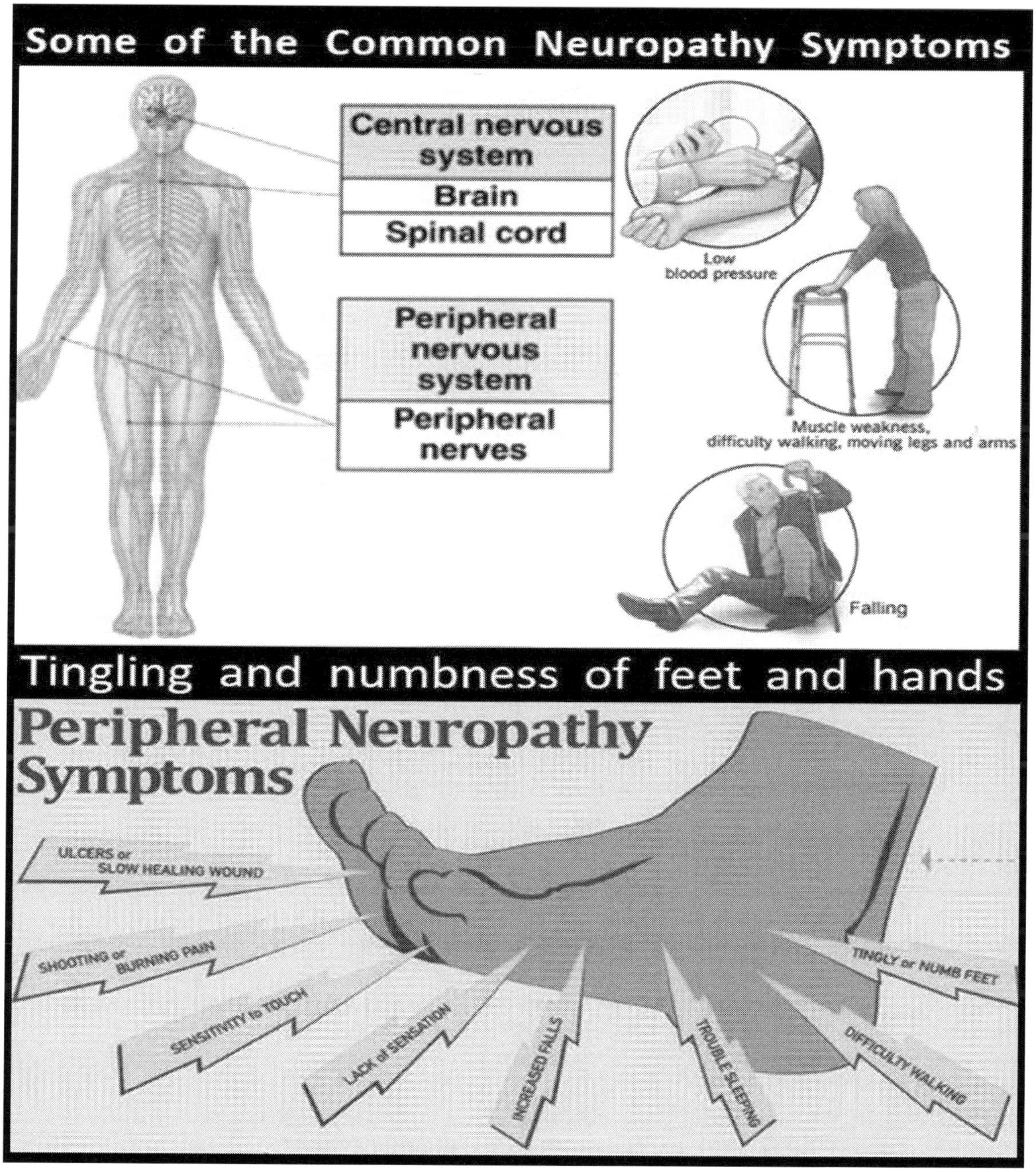

Case#4 Contaminated Faeces

Studies show that the coronavirus patient's faeces are also contaminated after 22 days taken from their stools instead of the usual 14 days retention period as in the case of other coronavirus studies conducted in SARS-CoV-1 in 2003 cases.

Faeces samples taken under microscope

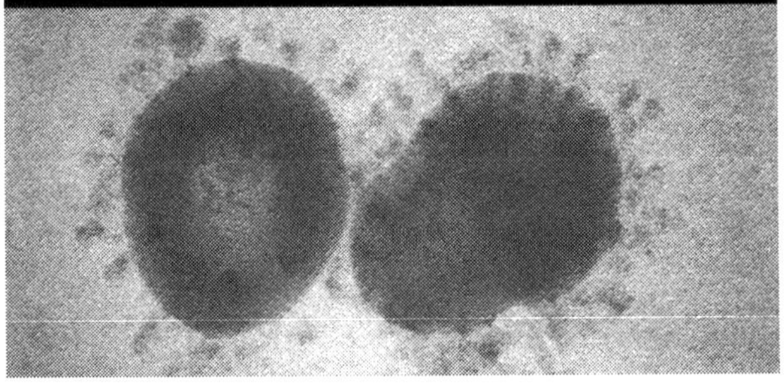

By using blood samples from COVID-19 patients, this test detects the antibodies whether they can neutralize the novel coronavirus and stopping the virus infecting cells.

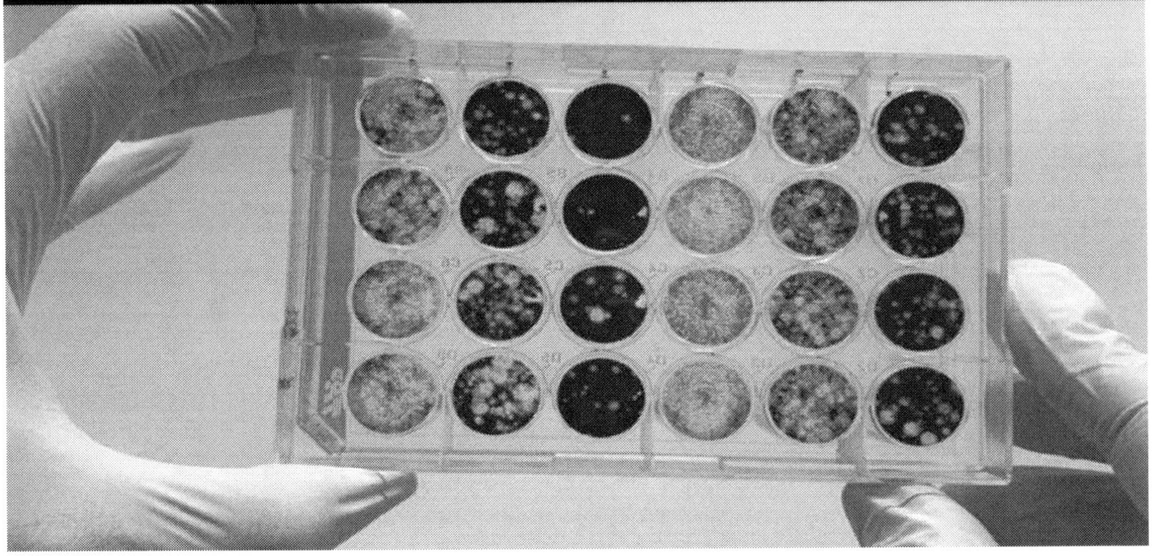

The viral RNA genetic material of the coronavirus from the respiratory tract, stool, blood serum and urine samples were extracted daily from the infected patients were sent to laboratory for detailing analysis.

Researchers and experts were equally surprised to find that there are also some other positive results found on their urine samples for coronavirus. Studies concluded that patients who are severely infected usually show a higher viral loads on germs count present in their samples as compared to those having mild infection cases.

With the viral loads' findings from the infected patients' samples taken, they hope they can become useful prognosis assessment, leading to future vaccine development of medical conditions to a solution of coronavirus treatments.

Case#5 SARS-CoV-2 Strains Mutate at Rapid Changes

Researchers from the Institute of Medical Research department had gathered laboratory evidences while doing virus isolation and virus culture to conclude that SARS-CoV-2 strains have another capabilities to mutate at rapid changes of 270 times.

As a result it creates some deadliness strains that ever seen before in medical history. That explains why there are existence of so many different types of virus strains coupled with different impacts that can affect so many different ethnic group differently in the world.

These mutations from the virus strains can evolve in so many combinations at one time.

Every time when a new mutation is created from the strains, it undergoes a substantially changing pattern on its pathogenicity (property of the disease) and virulence characteristics.

It directly alters the functional changes in the spike proteins that can enable certain mutations to form certain strains that are more deadly than the others can as a result severely damage the human immunity host cell.

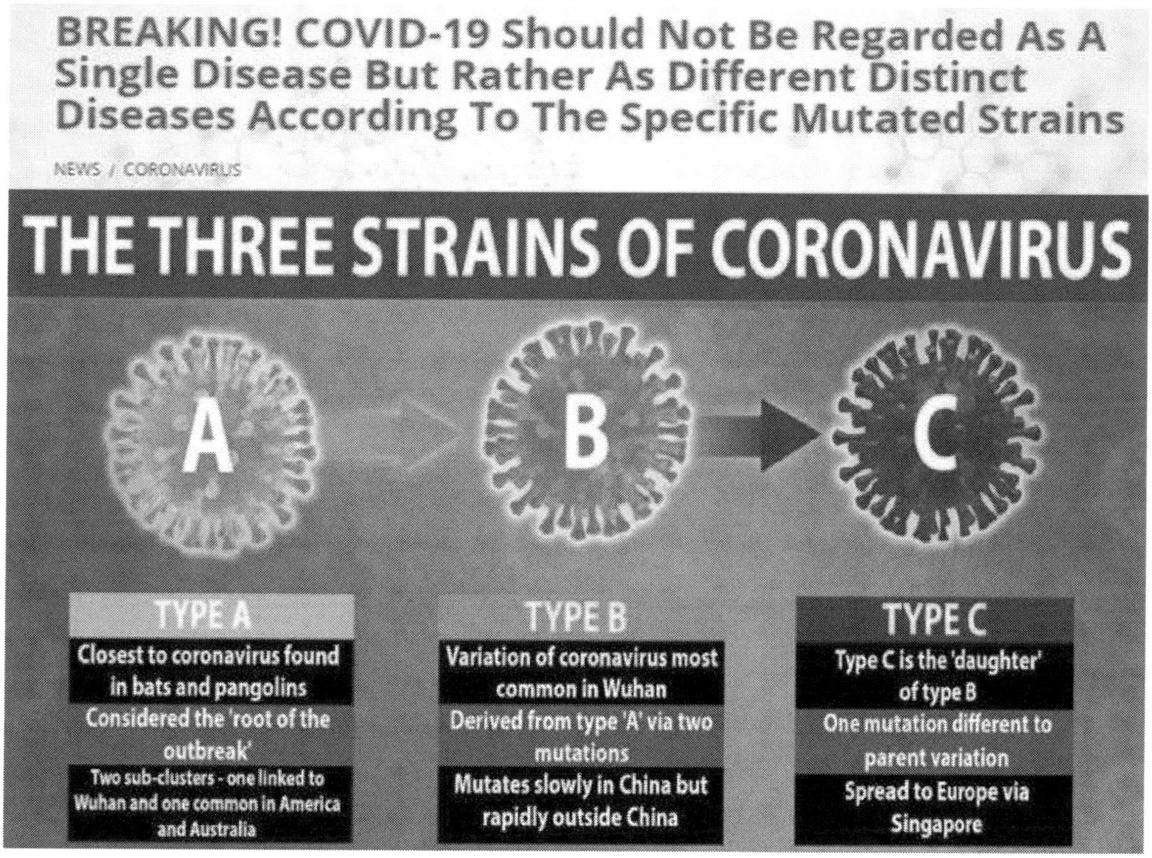

Case#6 Re-Infection of Coronavirus from Recovered Patient

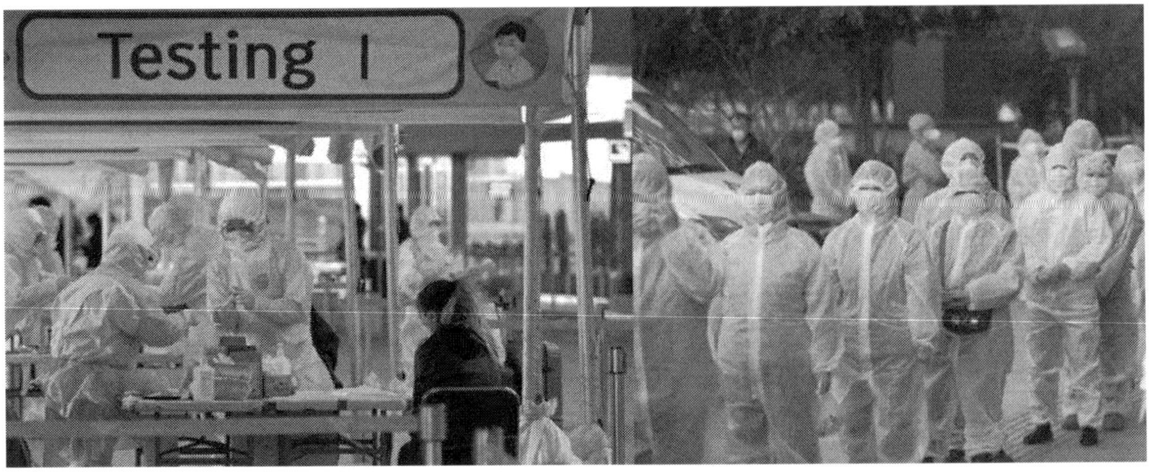

Throat Swab Test for COVID-19

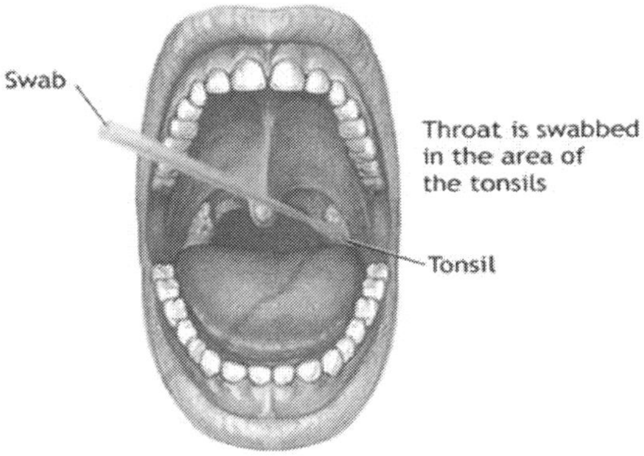

Nose Swab Test for COVID-19

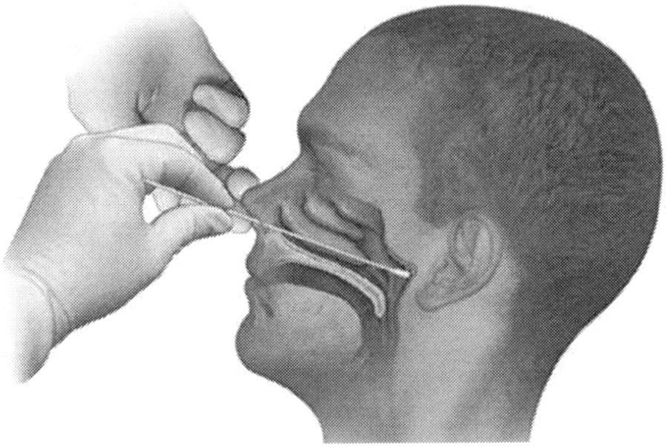

Recovered patients from coronavirus are not necessary becoming immune to the virus infections as re-infection can still be possible.

According to the Chinese investigations conducted experiments on recovered coronavirus patients, they discovered that discharged patients after returning back for COVID-19 test again, they are still tested positive for coronavirus even though they looked well and healthy and did not show any physical illness symptoms.

Generally, they look fine physically. Based on their analysis, the virus seem to have halted but then the viral RNA genetic code still remains dormant inside the patient immune system and can even leave it there for a period of unknown time.

There is no solid evidence to back up and proof that those recovered patients from COVID-19 are now able to self-develop its own antibodies and become immune from getting re-infected again the second time of reexposure to the virus transmission.

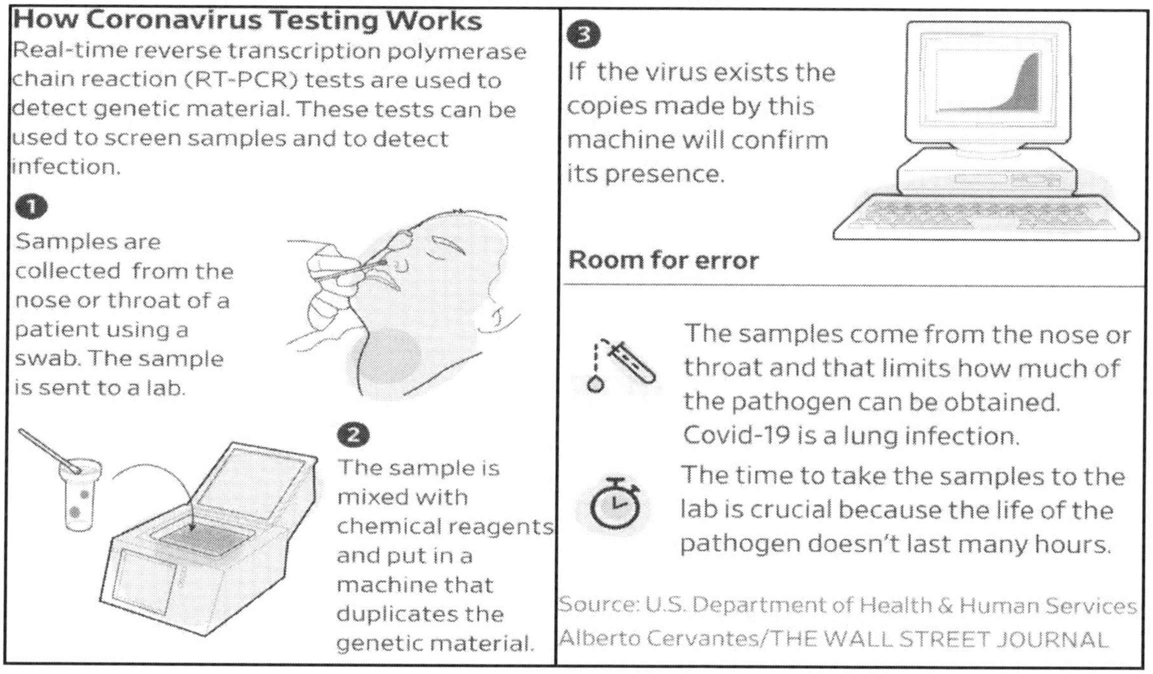

Other explanations for yielding such retesting positive results can be:

1. the chemicals used on the test kit's tissue paper
2. the virus had somehow been mutating in another form that is not being able to be identified by the coronavirus diagnostic test kit anymore

Some recommendations were proposed by government officials to issue an "immunity passport" to these recovered patients for easier identification from infected cases to allow them to resume work and travel freely. But, at this point in time, the recommendations were on-hold as the experts believe it is futile and incredibly risky until more understanding of the virus strains are being covered in this area.

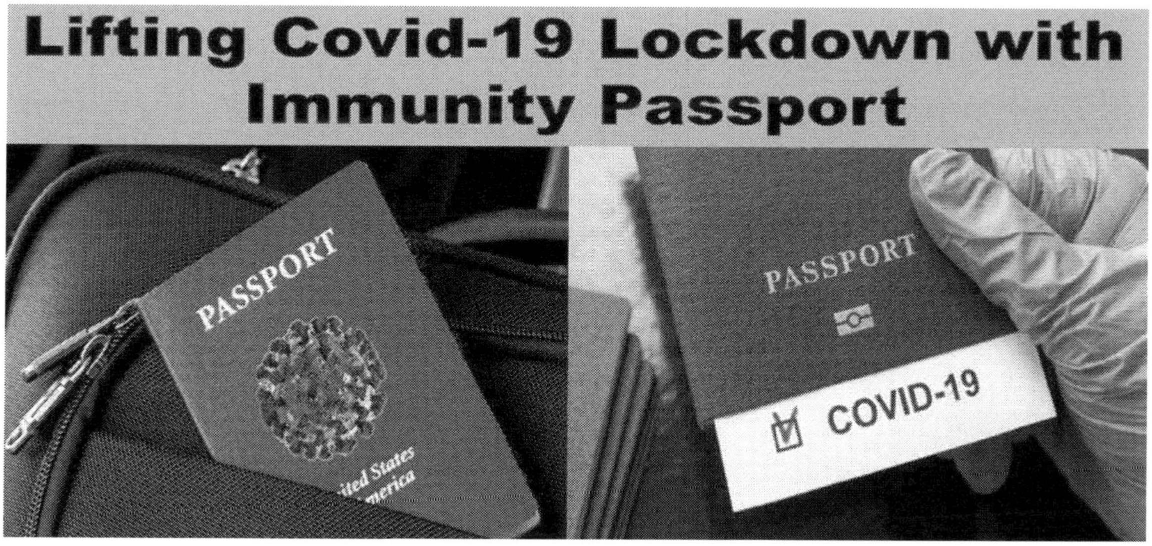

Microorganism Facts For Kids

Case#7 Vitamin Supplements to Boost Immune System

Advice recommend by the experts for those who are healthy to consume more Vitamins C and D to boost our self-health and immunity system to prevent coronavirus infection.

Good nutrition also plays an important part in supporting our human immunity functionality and development to fight any germs.

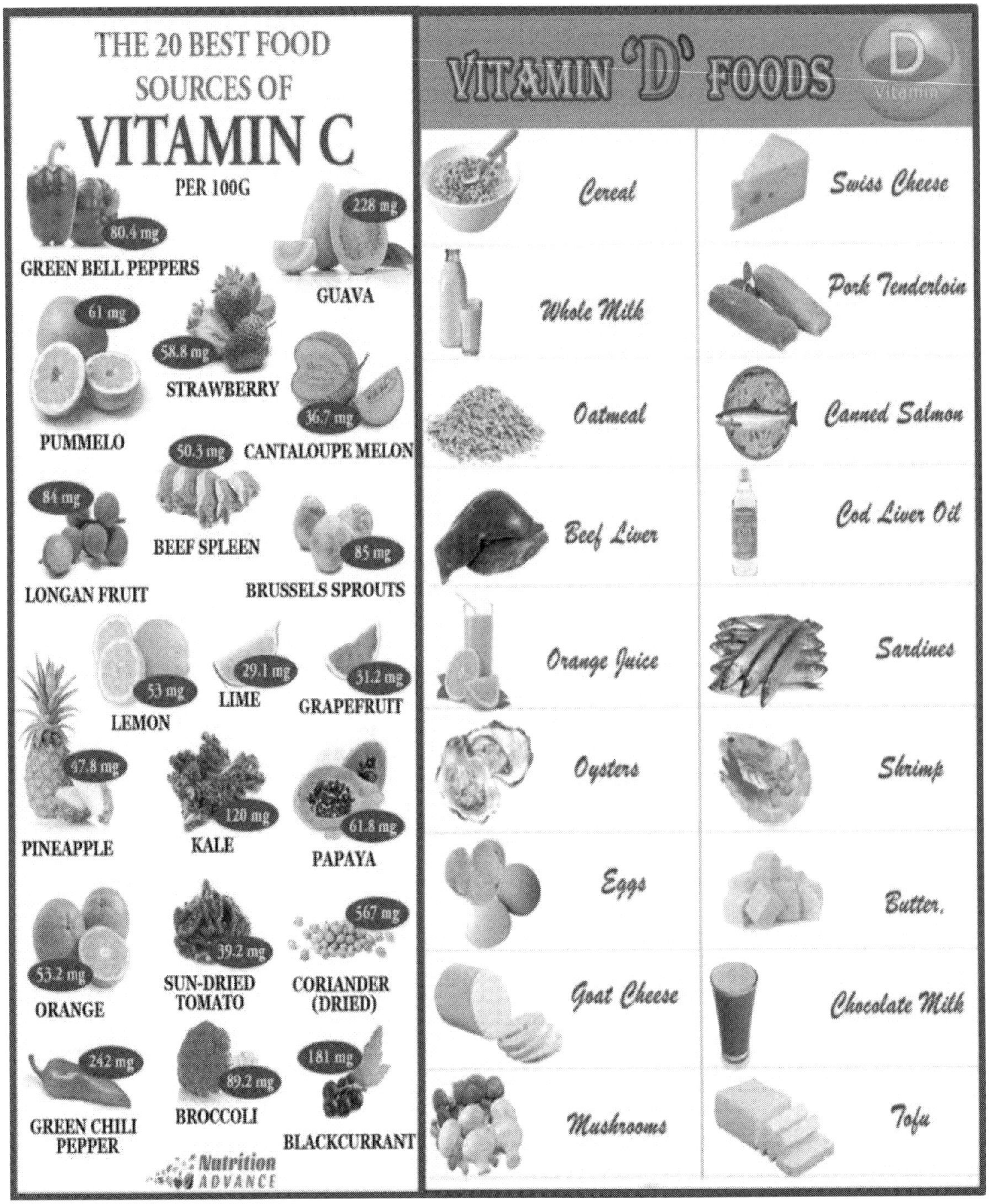

Case#8 Massive Heart Attack Sufferings

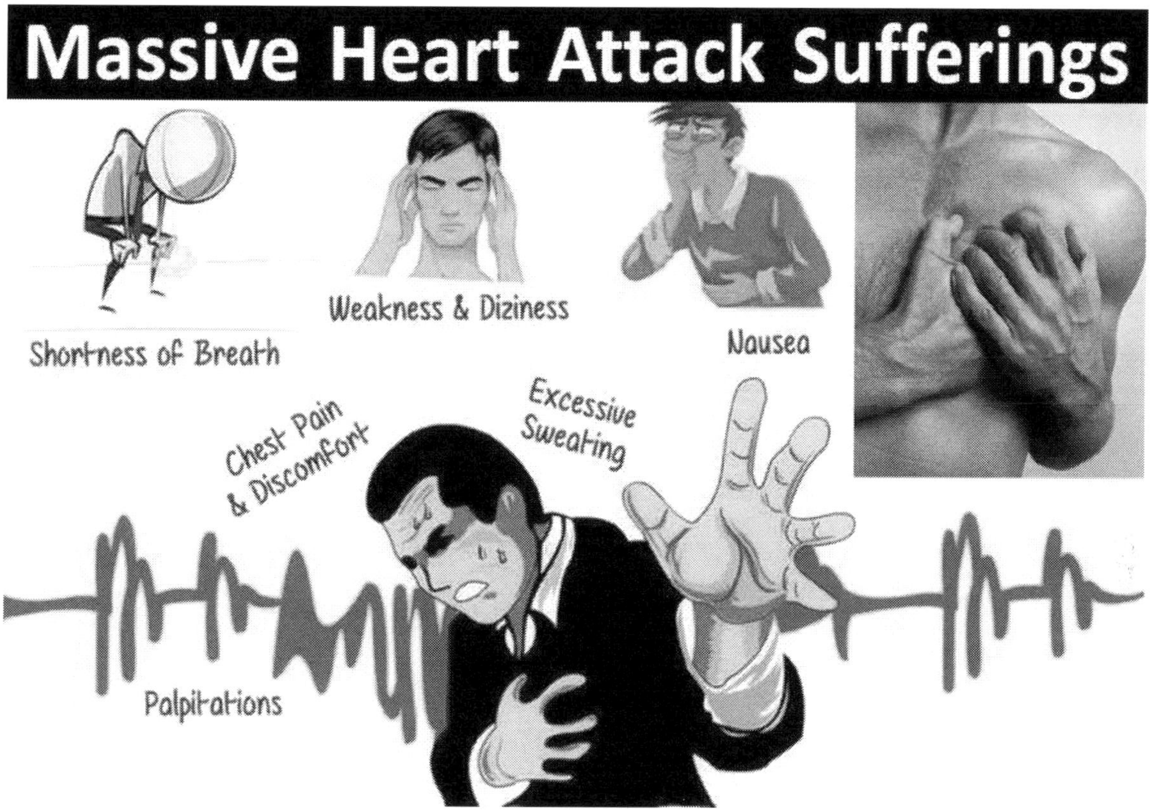

This is an extremely rare case that happened to one of the American elderly old lady at the age of 57 reported her death on 6 February 2020. She contracted the coronavirus infection and went into a series of massive heart attacks before her death.

Her autopsy report showed there were signs of viral infection in her heart, trachea, lungs and intestines throughout her whole body.

Before her death, she was initially checked in with just a simple flu-like symptoms. But, somehow her conditions deteriorated to the extent of suffering in great pains. Her heart muscles and other organs were found ruptured and ripped opened. No medical reasoning was able to explain such erratic and unusual virus behavioural attacks on humans.

COVID-19 behaves like one of the extremely rarest kind of viruses on Earth because of its mutation capability and ability to associate and combine with other viruses unlike bacteria. Viruses are really strange creatures indeed! Once they succeed to infiltrate into a human host cell, they start to eat it from inside. When they leave the cell, they are no longer a single cell but in millions. The old host cell is discarded and reduced nothing more than a garbage. This is their unique reproduction cycle.

Case#9 Positive Male Carriers of COVID-19 with Low Testosterone Level Correlate At Far Greater Risk of Dying

Clinicians have been unable to determine why men with virus-positive infections are facing higher risk of developing severe and lethal symptoms to death when comparing to women, independent of age. Studies conducted by researchers have seen male sex hormone testosterone cases admitted for intensive care had revealed that it play a vital role that correlates closely with the inflammatory cytokine.

Particularly in cases of low testosterone man, the situation becomes worst as the coronavirus triggers his body to produce large quantities of cytokines to storm and in return it releases more immune cells to aggressively fight against the pathogens.

In the ongoing process, it becomes disoriented and misdirected firing among the immune cells. As a result of such activity, a reversal backlash against itself occurs and the correlation of the inflammatory cytokine responses eventually leads to lethal outcome. This hyper-inflammatory condition itself gives rise to severe lung damage, acute respiratory distress syndrome (ARDS) and death.

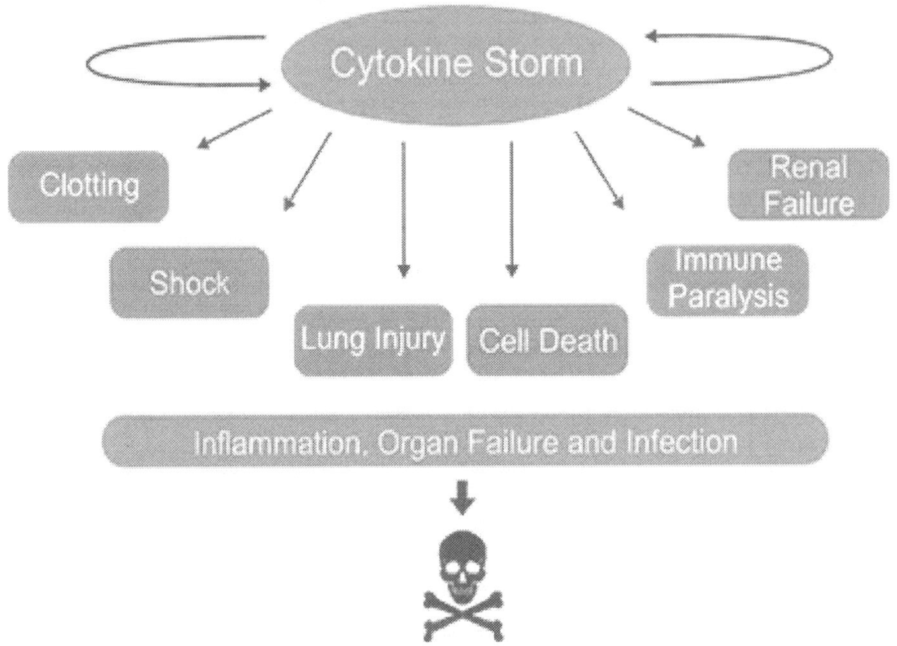

Generally, people with low testosterone dampen the impacts on the virus and induce more cytokine storms. When comparing to a healthy man with normal testosterone levels, cytokine storm will not be present and therefore he is more likely to survive from the coronavirus attack.

MICROORGANISM FACTS FOR KIDS

Testosterone plays an important key role factor in the regulation of our body's immunity responses. Henceforth, virus-positive men with low testosterone level must put on alert when admitted.

In general, testosterone function to produce bone tissues and also help to maintain bone volume. If a person inhibits a low testosterone level, there will be a reduction in his bone tissues volume that in turn makes the bones more susceptible to fractures as a result.

In addition, as age catches up in men especially from age 50 onwards, their testosterone production tends to slow down gradually and causing a reduction in his testicle size (nothing relating to cold temperatures) and his scrotum underneath will become softer than usual.

As a result, the amount of semen produced is reduced when ejaculating. He will often experience a significant lower sex drive too. Furthermore, a significant reduction to his muscle mass loss can gravely affect his functionality and strength of his muscles development. He can feel tired frequently and his body fat increases tremendously especially surrounding his breast areas due to lack of exercises and immobile muscles in a long run. Overall, he experiences erratic mood swings, lack of focus, irritability and depression behaviours all set in.

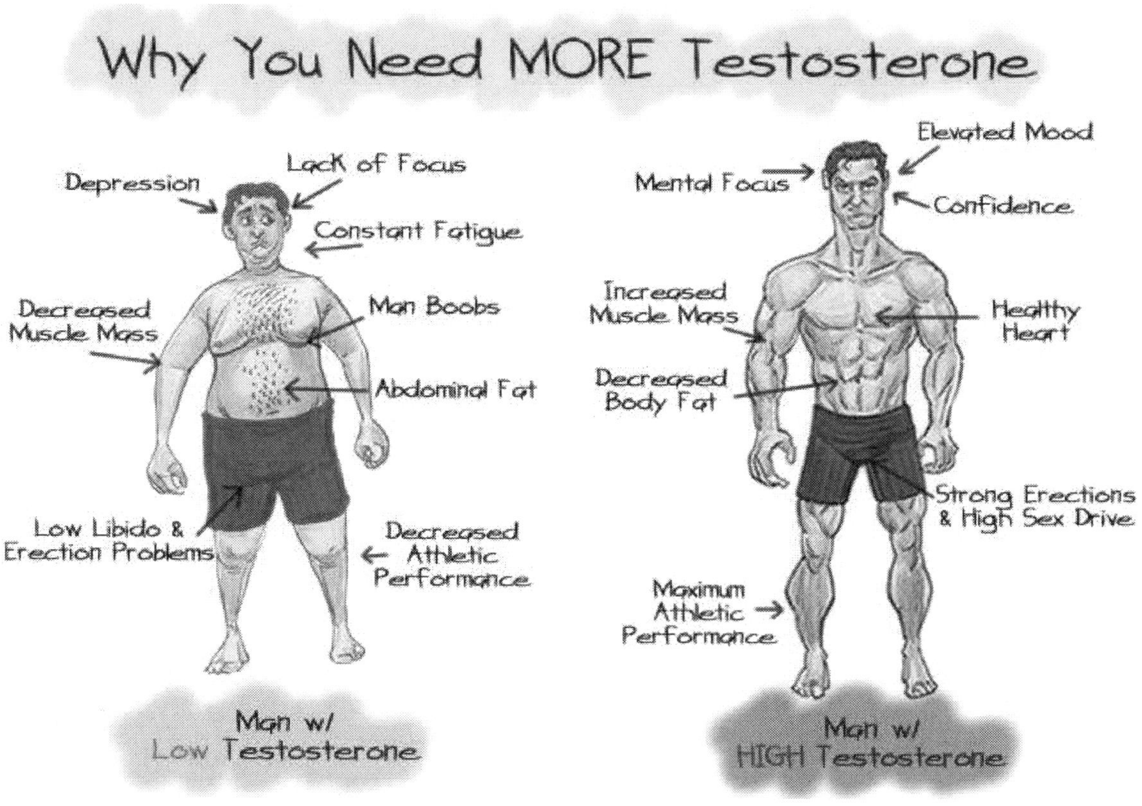

Microorganism Facts For Kids

Severe Safety Gear and Manpower Shortages

As the world is braving the fight against the deadly virus, lockdowns are inevitably unavoidable and uncertainty set in for everyone regardless of those working for people or running businesses. Businesses are finding hard to sustain its operations. Some went bust, filing for bankruptcy or companies are overseeing to implement several cost-containment measures such as salary reduction and short work week, putting in hiring freezes and making it discretionary spending cuts across all departments from "top to the bottom" management levels due to a decline in customer volume base caused by the COVID-19 pandemic.

Presented with this outcome, nation leaders are establishing community schemes to help people to defray the living cost and at the same time to help cushioning and supporting local businesses in this trying times to minimise layoffs and urging firms to preserve jobs.

On the other hand, healthcare sectors are facing severe manpower shortages, hospital beds, PPE accessories and equipment as many people are admitted for COVID-19 swab testing and others for COVID-19 related conditions amid the pandemic.

Hospitals are busy tackling on the front lines of the outbreak. More additional tents and isolation facilities are being put up outside the hospital complex to complement the shortage of hospital beddings and wards.

China coronavirus: crowds and confusion on the hospital front lines of outbreak

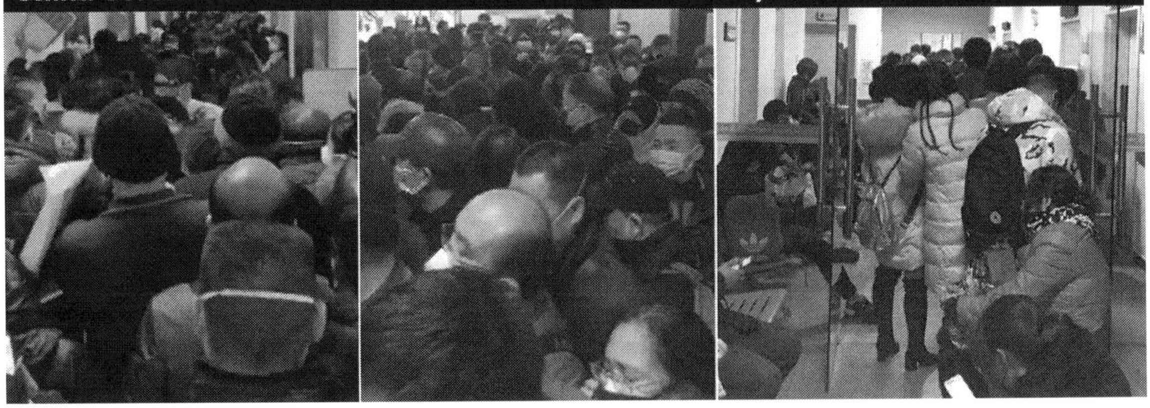

In hospitals, doctors and nurses are rushing to incubate and rescue the infected patients in the midst of ventilators shortage. In some critical instances of saving livers, doctors face a tough decision to make as to whom to rescue first between the young and the elderly due to severe ventilator shortages in hospitals to assist patients to breathe on its own.

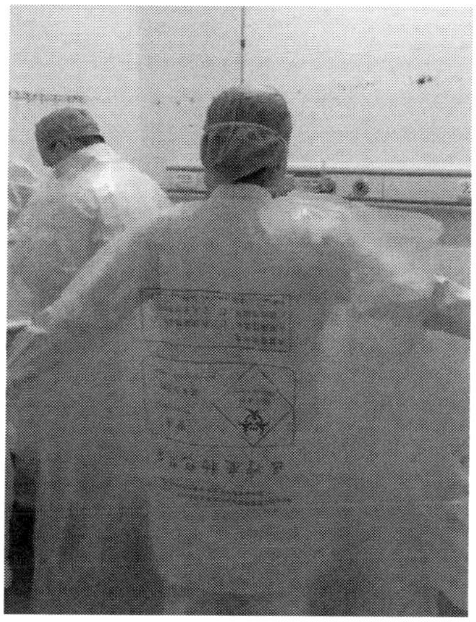

Medical workers are pleading for supplies of PPE gears. The dire shortages of PPE supplies cause many to resort and improvise their own protective coverings by turning to tapes for patching up their battered protective face masks, reusing their googles repeatedly time and again, wrapping their shoes over with some plastic bags in the lack of specialised coverings at hospitals.

Some even use diver snorkelling as a substitute to N95 mask even it does not offer any protection against viruses.

Doctors are seen using improvised gears made from home-made face masks and nursing attires from trash bin bags, sounding off that the nationwide hospitals are in chronic shortages of safety gear and equipment such as masks, goggles, gowns and respirators etc. Some went to the extent of scouring from the hardware stores to get hold of any protective masks and googles for replacements in hospital urgent needs.

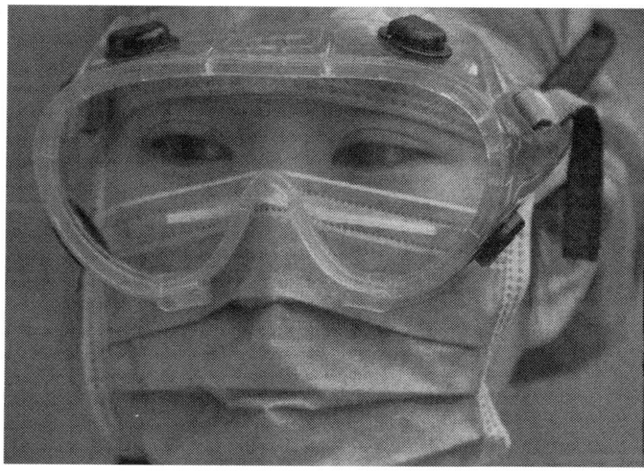

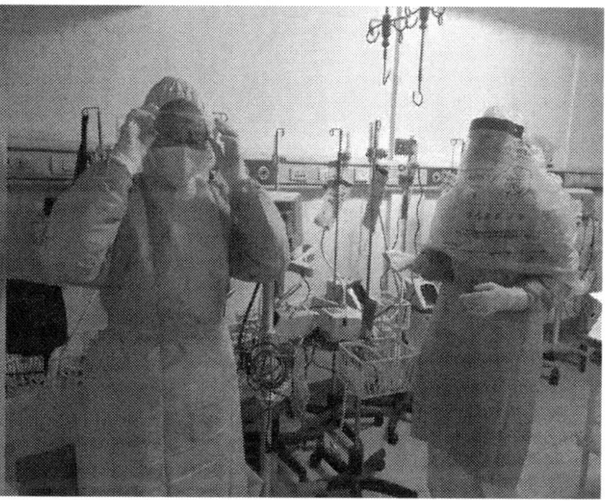

The confrontation of the viral epidemic outbreak coupled with barely sufficient supply of protective equipment (PPE) had made the frontline workers vulnerable at the mercy of the coronavirus infection.

Some medical workers including doctors and nurses alike were tested COVID-19 positive. Others were unfortunately had to sacrifice their noble lives for others to live on. During this pandemic handling situations, their selfishness and heroic acts really make us feel proud for them and we lament together with the rest of the staffs over their sacrificial loss too regardless of nationality, political affiliation, race, colour or gender.

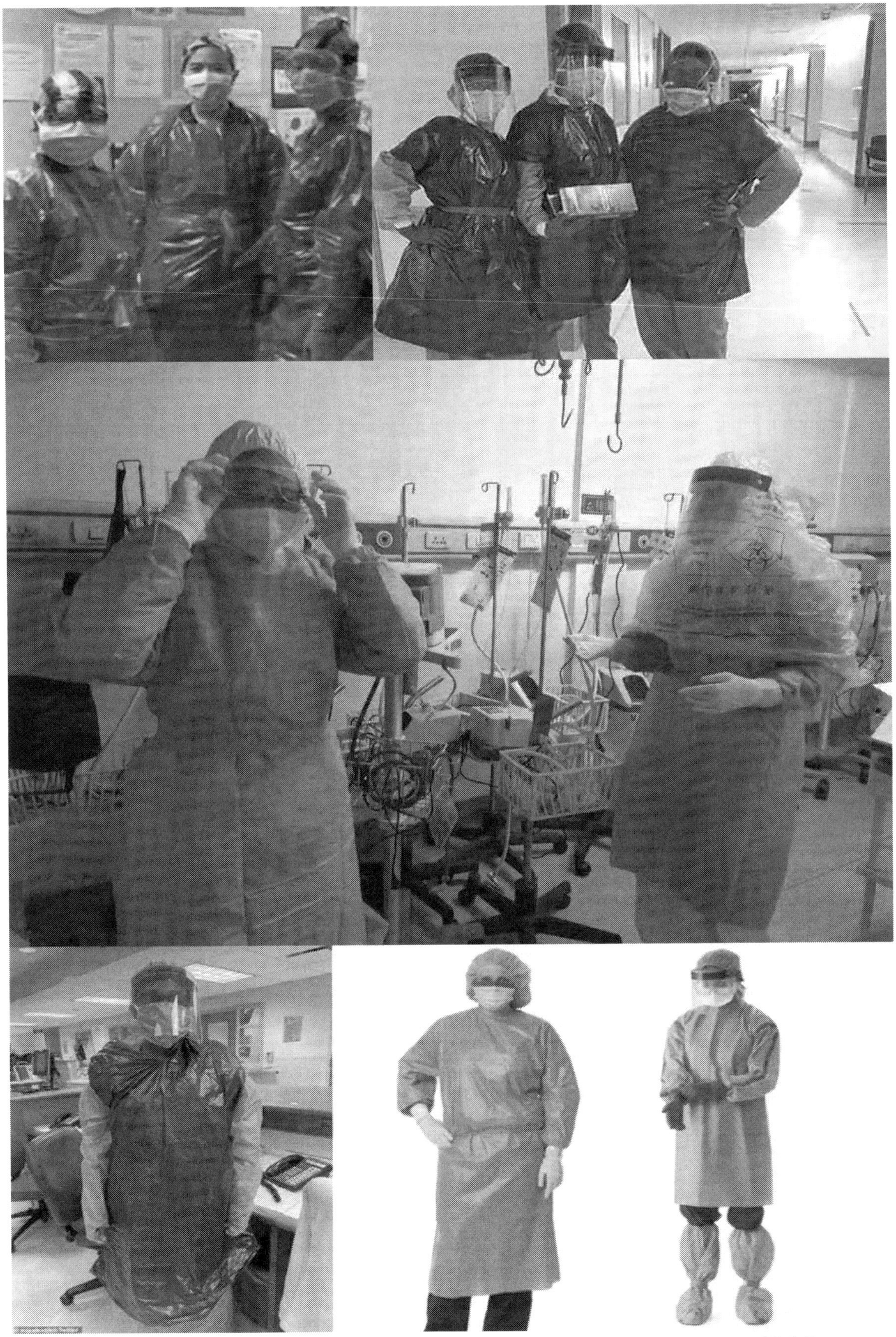

MICROORGANISM FACTS FOR KIDS

Many touching stories were shared publicly on Instagram and Facebook social media by the frontliners. Sad sobbing stories were revealed that their elderly volunteered to give up their lives for the young ones to survive in face of the chronic ventilator shortages in the hospital.

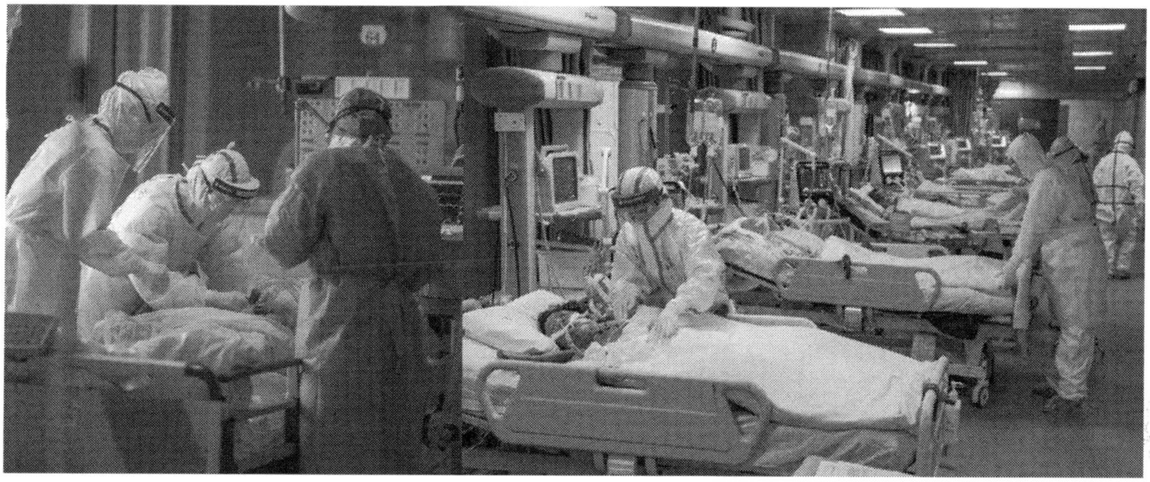

"I'm so scared!" said one of the nurses who cried tearfully in front of the social media. Some couldn't take the pressure and tender their resignation, "The chaos and the lack of protective equipment. Patients keep coming in like waves and we are not getting the kind of support we need as we are directly exposing ourselves to the positive COVID-19 patients daily. I want to give up saving these people!"

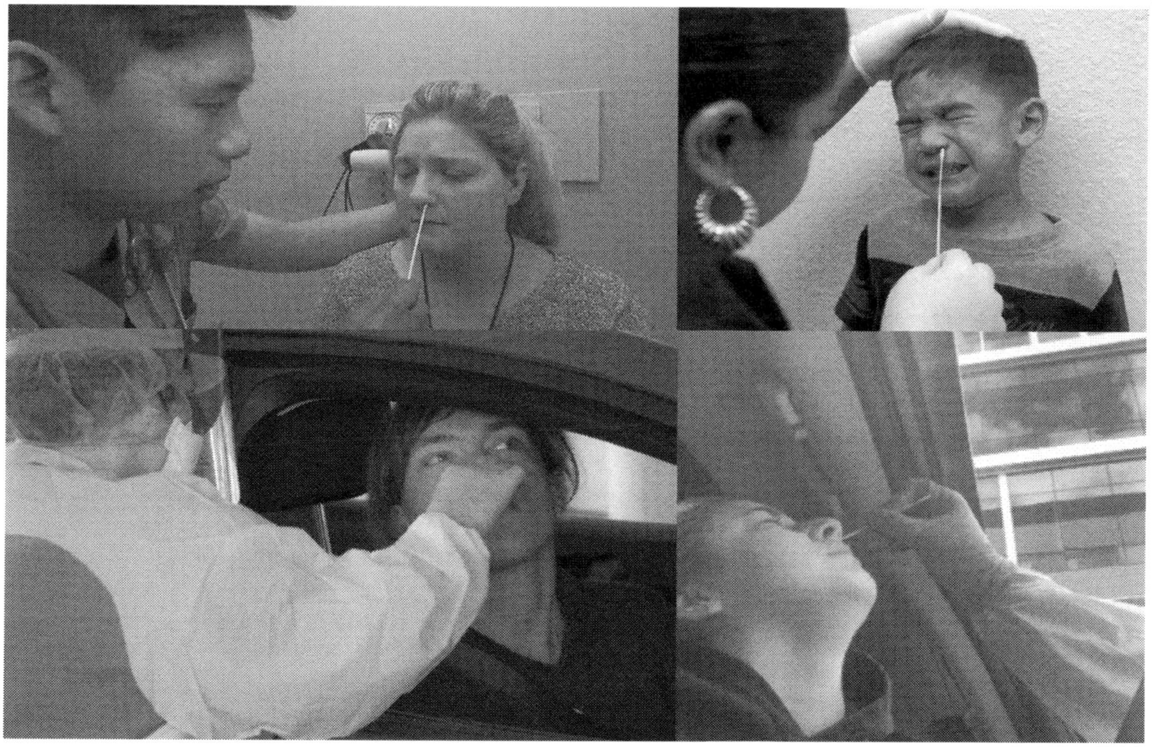

Microorganism Facts For Kids

COVID-19 Swab Test Kits

Antibody tests can detect the presence of antibodies in the blood that bind to the coronavirus that causes COVID-19. As such, antibody tests are the key to slowing down the coronavirus infection rate.

The concept of COVID-19 test kit is similar to the way the pregnancy test kit works.

In COVID-19 test kit, the test paper strip is coated with a monoclonal antibodies that is bonded with some viral proteins and then dips into a certain solution containing the patient sample nanoparticles.

The outcome of the result will be known soon in a couple of 30 minutes later upon which a coloured indicator appears and shows up on the paper strip to decide whether the person gets COVID-19 or not.

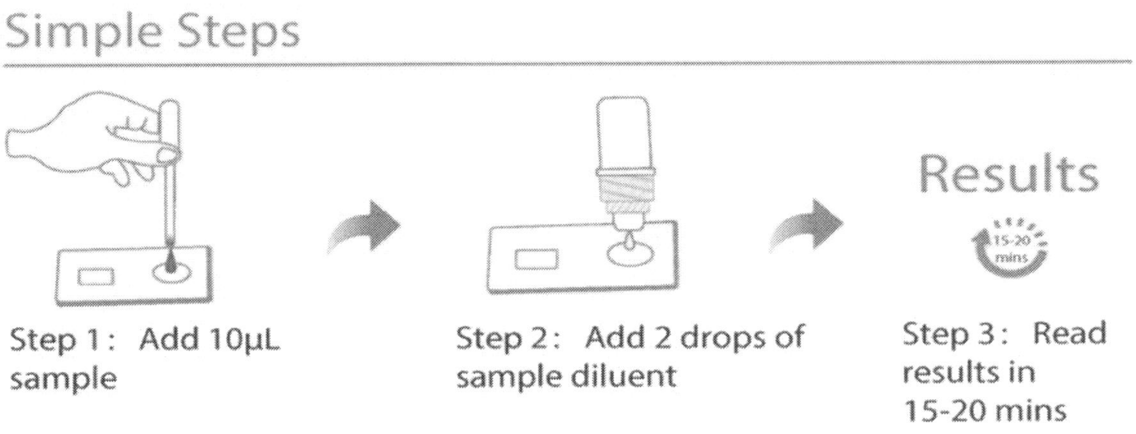

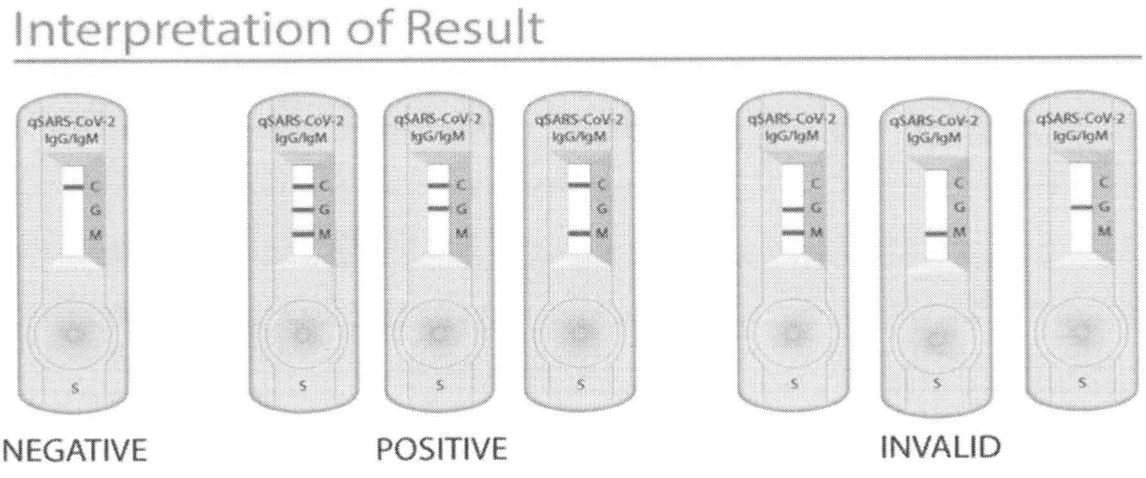

MICROORGANISM FACTS FOR KIDS

United and Togetherness We Fight the Virus

Let us do our part and together we can curb it by stemming out the spread of the coronavirus!

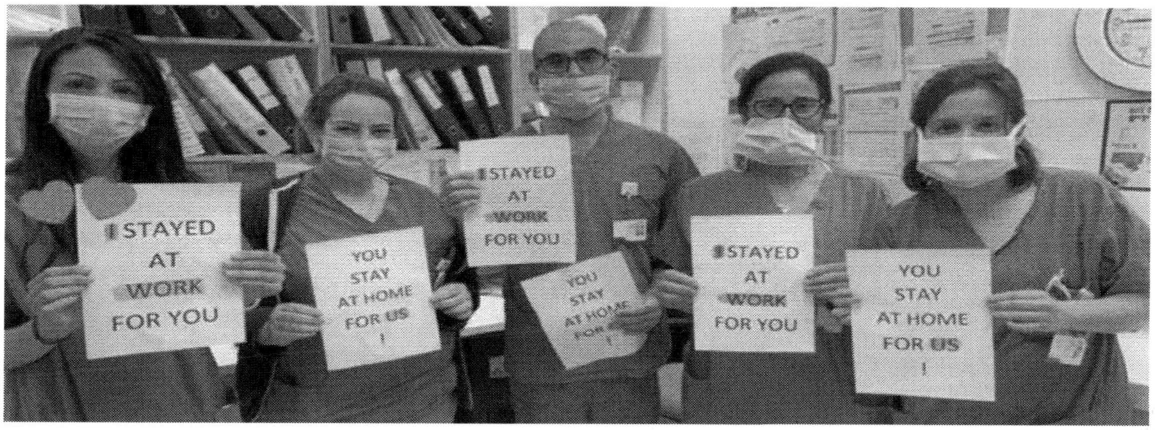

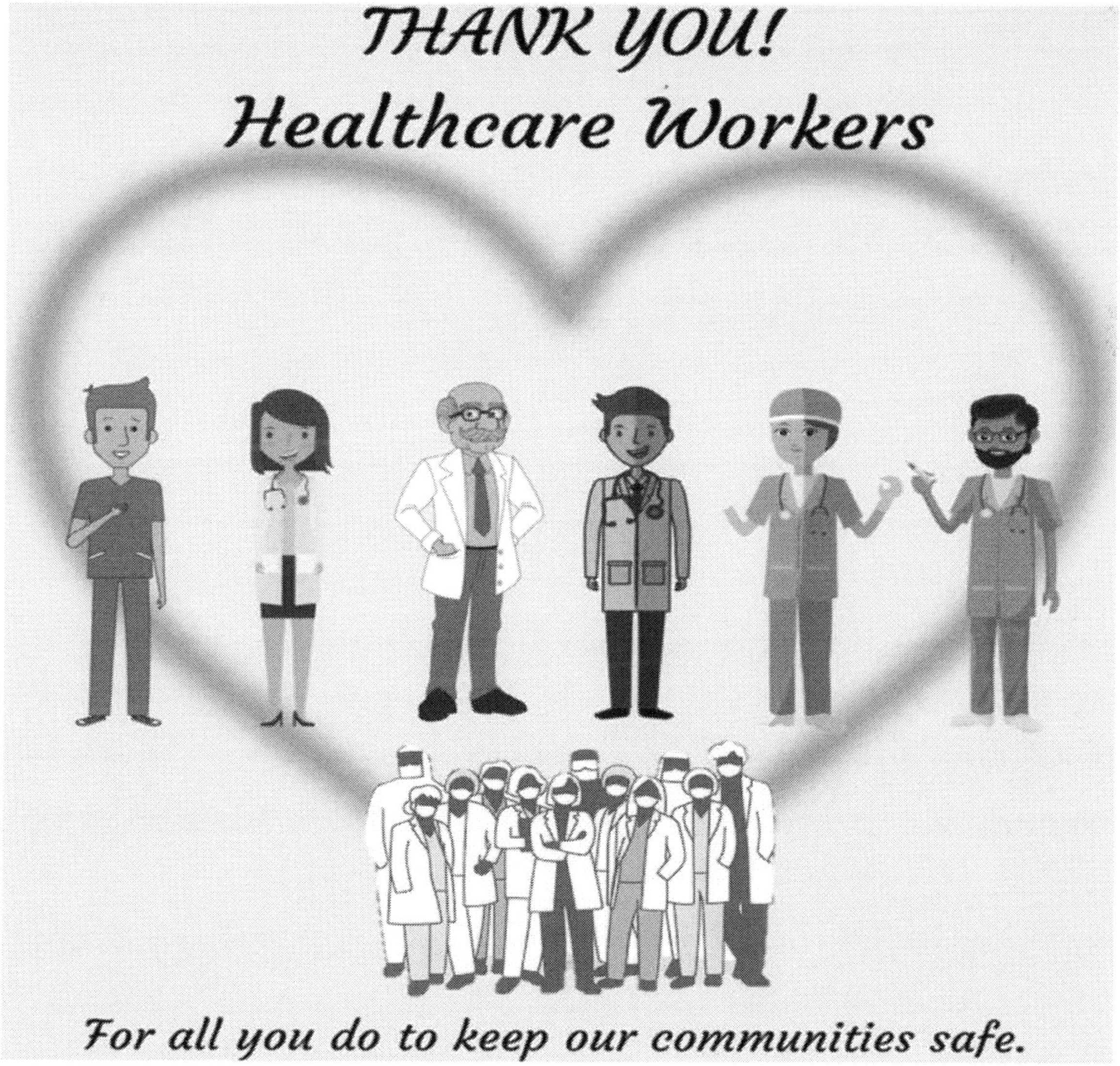

China, Wuhan Bans Wild Animals Consumption

Published by MarketWatch news on 23 May 2020, China enforce a mandatory ban on consumption of its exotic meat at its wet markets trading in Wuhan, the epicentre coronavirus outbreak in Hubei province.

Targeting on wild animals such as lion, tiger, snake, peacock and pangolin etc. are strictly to be taken out from the food menu after the municipal Chinese government made official announcement that the new legislation come into immediate force to ban, breed, hunt and consumption of these wild animals as part of the national campaign to halt the sale and consumption of exotic meats in wet markets that was blamed by many to have spawned the coronavirus diseases on current pandemic situation. This new law will be in force for five years and will be reviewed again when the term ends.

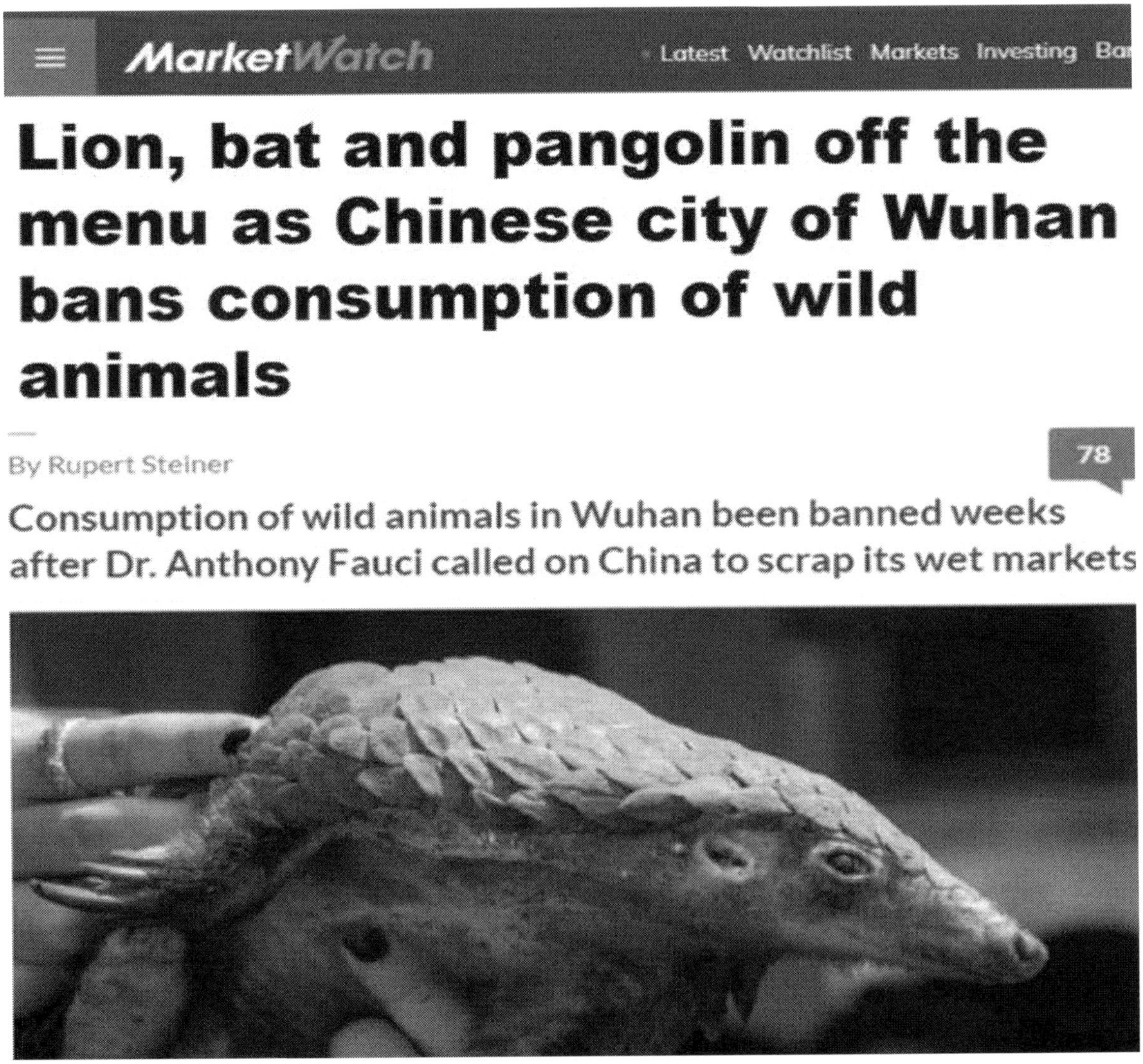
MarketWatch · Latest Watchlist Markets Investing Ba

Lion, bat and pangolin off the menu as Chinese city of Wuhan bans consumption of wild animals

By Rupert Steiner

78

Consumption of wild animals in Wuhan been banned weeks after Dr. Anthony Fauci called on China to scrap its wet markets

Microorganism Facts For Kids

The Virus Battling of the Poor Nation Sickness

Some predicted that there is going to have a future widespread coronavirus infection in Africa and other poorer regions where their healthcare systems are less developed and in need of great funding support and medical supplies in the wake of the virus pandemic threats.

Many nations depend on the poor nations like Africa, Yemen, South Sudan, Venezuela, Zimbabwe, Cameroon, Afghanistan, Haiti, Nigeria etc. to grow agricultures and crops for their global exports. By depriving this financial support and medical supplies, it can create an exponential spike in its infections spread swiftly across these continents.

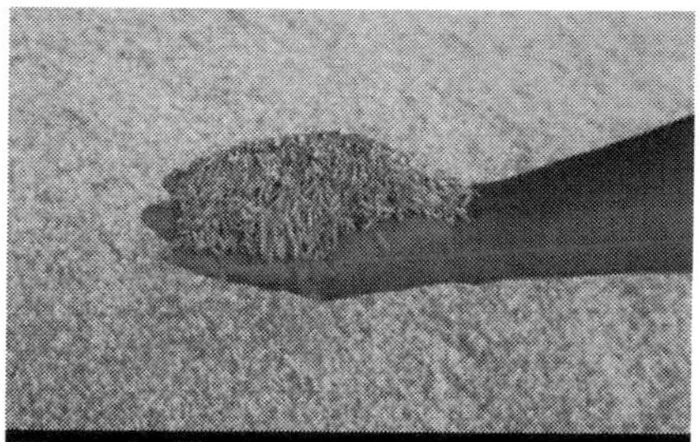

Food Shortages Expected to Affect One Billion People

As a result, the infection spreads bring the whole world into a severe scarcity of food shortages. Chaotic and erratic situations become worse. Prices of food stuffs and groceries globally will have immediate shock of steep increase, resulting panic fears over food crisis. Every nation experience anxiety fears and starts to stock up everything in anticipation of its global severe shortages and steep prices on all goods.

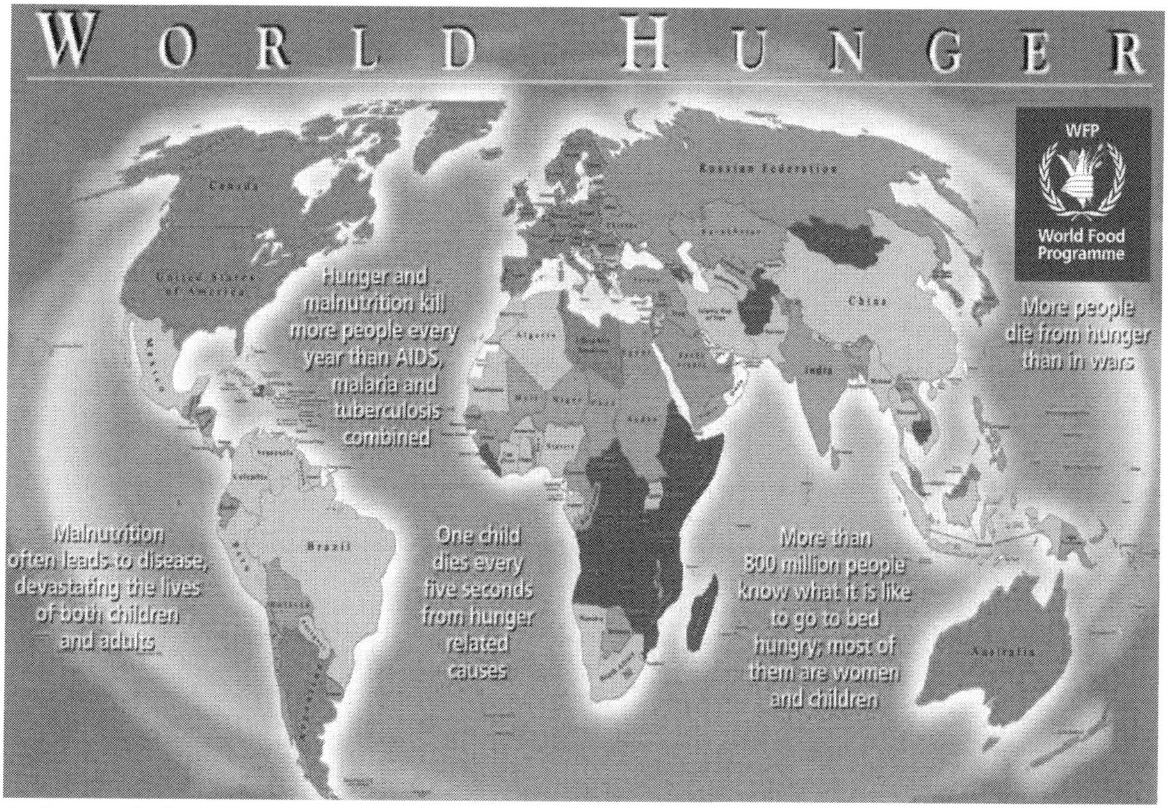

Market Analysis in COVID-19

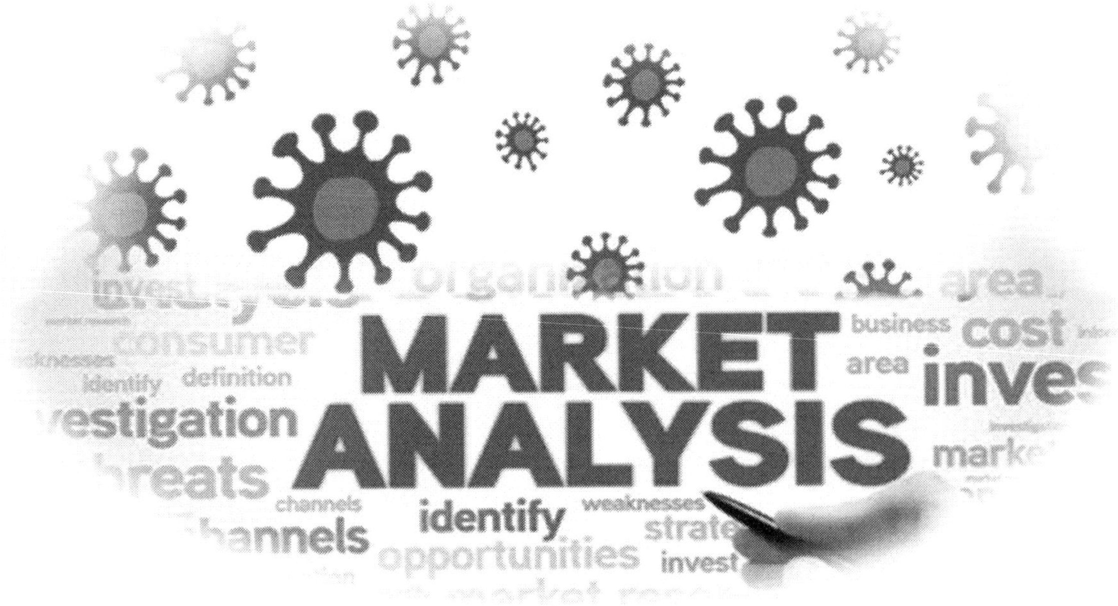

With Corona Virus Disease 2019, COVID-19, the whole world is putting up a fierce fight to the dual COVID pandemic. This entails towards health and economic pandemic that had impacted trillions of dollars of revenues from country reserves to help businesses to stay afloat and preserve jobs and preventing people from losing jobs.

But still, it doesn't seem to work as restaurants have been filing for bankruptcy and many more businesses are at risk too as consumer patterns are no longer having the same spending and buying behaviour like it was before the pandemic.

Some Food & Beverages outlet had been crippled and struggling with weak traffic even after lockdown phases have been lifted gradually. Fresh dine-in restrictions were mandatory adhered to and everyone is on fears of the next wave of COVID-19 infections. Crowds are not coming back at all and running a business is like piling up debts and sky-high rentals. Many of them are on their shoestring budget now to cut costs as no one can foresee what lies ahead in the coming years.

Poverty in Southeast Asia is going to surge in "socio-economic crisis" crippled by the COVID-19 pandemic and threatens to destroy livelihood and pushing many families into poverty, reversing decades of poverty reduction if there is no stimulus measures and medical support assistance render to save the situation.

MICROORGANISM FACTS FOR KIDS

1. Aviation, Travel and Tourism

People are not making travel plans. Airlines have already been cutting down flights and offered ridiculous flight rates to get people to fly again. But, people still hardly want to fly for fear of getting infected.

2. Retailing and eCommerce

Consumers' confidence drops drastically as many prefer to stay indoors at this crisis. Some F&B businesses and all other non-essential services are not opening up even lockdown phase is lifted as crowd is not coming as it was before. Almost, many are shutting down and turning to web-based businesses instead of the usual way of brick and mortar store. Only supermarket stores, markets and essential services are allowed to operate but public health preventive measures must still continue to be strictly followed. Increasingly enforcement officers are walking round the ground to take stern action against individuals, business owners or entities who intentionally flout the orders and requirements.

Nevertheless, eCommerce digital businesses are thriving as more people are now staying at home placing more online orders for groceries and food delivering.

3. Financial and Banking

Newly start-up companies have difficulties seeking funds from Venture Capitalist, bringing fewer investments in the stock market crash as the pandemic poses a biggest threat to the global economy and financial markets. Credit landing facility and mortgage loan are being tightened by banks in anticipating for the worst economy ahead.

U.S. Federal Reserve has implemented a deep cut in interest rates across the world to help and stabilise the world economy market in effect of the global depression that had caused job losses and business unsustainability.

4. Hyperlocal Marketing Services (Delivery Businesses)

Hyperlocal Delivery Company for examples Deliveroo and GrabFood are thriving. They are quick to react to the market downturn and are offering options for their customers to either choose a contact-less delivery or have the items delivered directly to the doorstep by their riders. Doorstep delivery services for food, medicine, grocery, and packages to name a few are gaining better ground in the wake of the pandemic crisis.

5. Recreation

Entertainment centers like movie theatres, pubs and art galleries are shutting down and not allowed to operate until further notice by the authorities due to a high risk of a large social gatherings that can bring in the means of the virus transmission spread.

6. Education

Lesser or simply none of the oversea students are willing to travel out of their country to pursue their studies elsewhere now at this national pandemic.

Zoom, a modern enterprise video communication solution using cloud technology, saw a surge of users globally deploying it for businesses and school telecommuting purposes as many working people are adhering to staying at home orders and schools are moving children towards home based learning to remain safe.

VPN, virtual private network, routing from internet broadband had seen a surge in its internet connectivity linkage globally by statutory board.

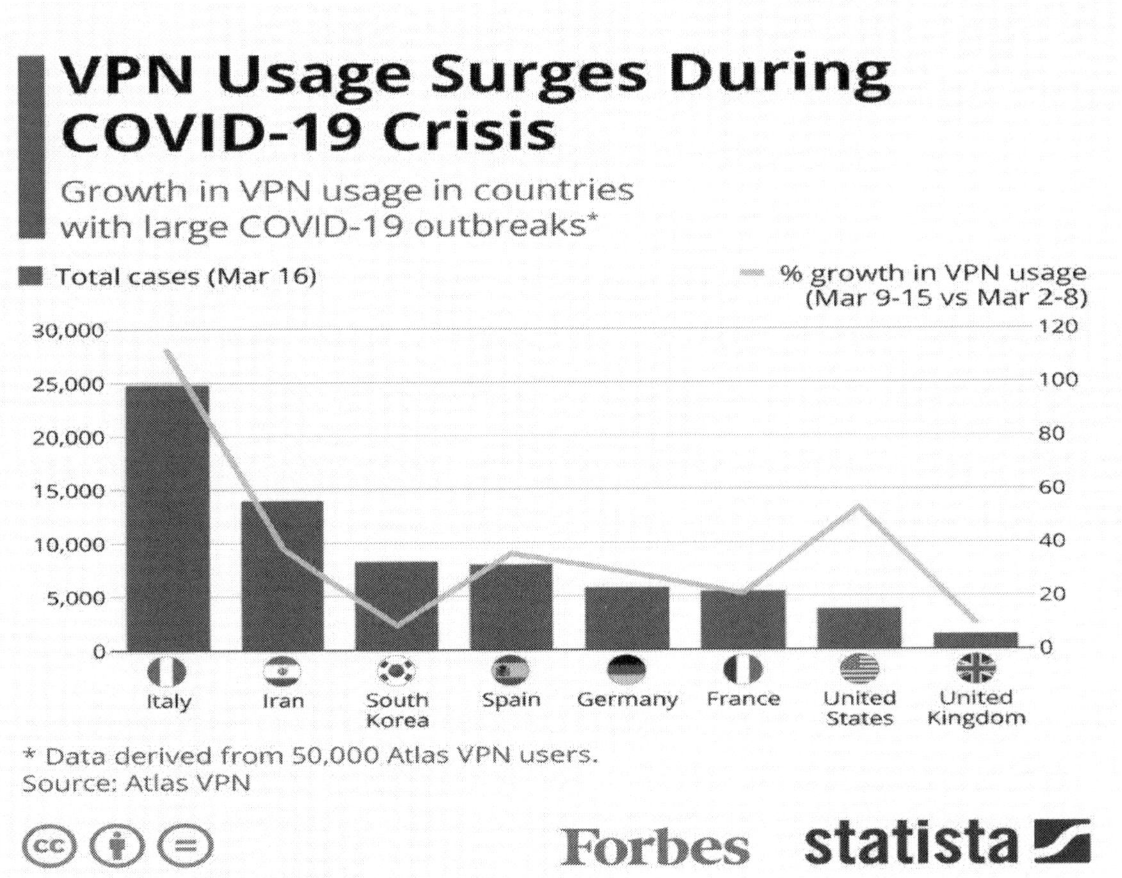

Business Imperatives and Insights

HOSPITALITY, TOURISM

Industry Size
Hotels - ₹**37,000-39,000 cr**
Tourism - ₹**18 lakh cr**
Total Employees: **40 million**

CORONA IMPACT

1] Tourism body expects **1.2 million** direct job losses

2] Ancillary industries like logistics will also take a severe hit

3] Hotelivate estimates revenue loss at $1.3-1.55 billion (₹9,600-11,400 cr) in short term, **27-32% drop** over last year

4] 15-25% casual/contract employees to suffer first blow

5] Indians make up 10% of global cruise liner staff; most may lose jobs

Industry View: Achin Khanna, managing partner, Hotelivate: A large mass of skilled manpower will be scrounging for opportunities... that is a serious crisis

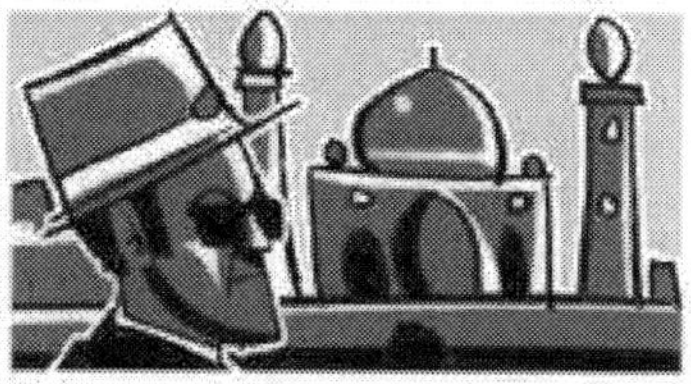

RESTAURANTS

Industry Size: ₹**4.2 lakh crore**
Total Employees: **7.3 million**

CORONA IMPACT

1] **15-20%** job losses likely (as of now)

2] Impact could be bigger

Industry View: Anurag Katriar, president, NRAI: The outbreak has severely impacted F&B industry... this business has high fixed operating costs

AVIATION

Industry Size: ₹**2.22 lakh cr**
Total Employees: **350,000**

CORONA IMPACT

1] Consultant Capa estimates **$600 m** (₹4,200 cr) loss in April-June for private carriers

2] If crisis continues, **150 aircraft** may be grounded

3] So far, no talk of job losses, but pressure will increase if traffic remains thin

4] AI has cut allowances, layover times

5] GoAir has asked employees to go on rotational leave without pay

Industry View: SK Singh, ED (finance), Air India: Keeping in view company financials... need to contain costs... globally, airlines are taking steps...

RETAIL

Industry Size: ₹**59 lakh crore**
Total Employees: **46 million**

CORONA IMPACT

1] Severe setback if crisis persists for three months

2] **11 million** (25%) jobs may be lost

Industry View: Kumar Rajagopalan, CEO, Retailers Association of India: Without govt help, millions may lose jobs

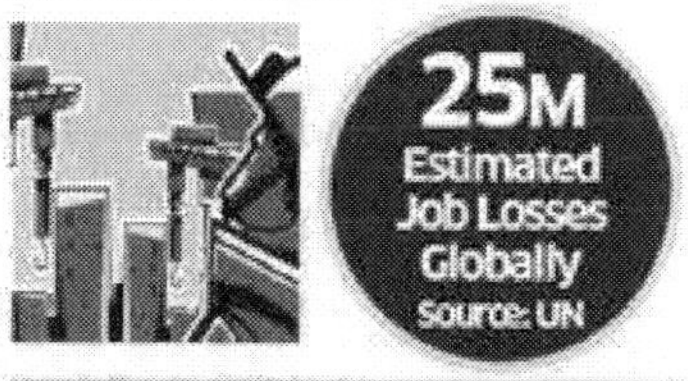

REAL ESTATE

Industry size: ₹**13.32 lakh cr**
2nd-largest employer after agri

CORONA IMPACT

1] Economic slump had already wiped away nearly 20% jobs

2] Outbreak will make it worse, leading to almost **35% job losses**

Industry View: Niranjan Hiranandani, president (national), Naredco: Outbreak will lead to volatility and turn positive net-worth firms into NPAs. This will lead to value erosion and job losses

RIDE-HAILING

Industry Size: ₹**11.84 lakh cr**
Total Employees: **5 m** driver-partners (largely Ola, Uber)

CORONA IMPACT

1] Demand down by **40-50%**

2] Driver-partners' earnings to be hit

Industry View: Pravin Agarwala, cofounder of BetterPlace: Though a few companies have agreed to give the basic payout – around ₹12,000-₹14,000 a mth – most drivers rely heavily on incentives

ONLINE FOOD DELIVERY

Industry Size: ₹**48,000 crore**
Total Employees: **500,000 (Flexi-jobs)**, as per internal estimates by Swiggy & Zomato

CORONA IMPACT

1] No immediate job loss

2] Income has **dipped 20%** on average for delivery partners

Industry View: Harsha Razdan, partner, KPMG India: Consumption will get curtailed or reduced. Firms that have equipped staff with remote working resources will be better off

ECOMMERCE

Industry Size: ₹**22.7 lakh cr** (as per RedSeer Consulting)
Total Employees: **6.1 m** (as per Indian Staffing Federation)

CORONA IMPACT

1] Online shopping has gone up, so no immediate impact

2] If crisis persists and demand sinks, **20-30% job losses** likely

Industry View: Suchita Dutta, ED, Indian Staffing Federation: No one has plans to downsize immediately... organisations are still trying to assess the situation

CINEMA, ENTERTAINMENT

Industry Size: ₹**1.82 lakh cr**
Total Employees: **7-8 m**

CORONA IMPACT

1] Contract, freelance employees most vulnerable

2] No job cuts being discussed yet

3] Pressure to mount if crisis continues

Industry View: Siddharth Jain, owner & director, Inox Leisure: If this continues into April and May, I shudder to even think about it. Rationalisation of salaries or a haircut at senior level may be needed

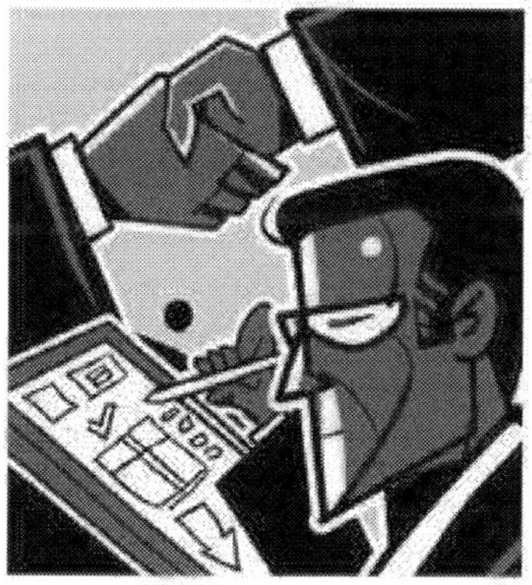

TEMP STAFFING

Industry Size: ₹**44,400 crore**
Total Employees: **4.1 million** in 2019 (as per Indian Staffing Federation)

CORONA IMPACT

1] Face-to-face interviews out, online in

2] Tech talent demand freezing up

3] Those who can't work from home to be hit

4] **Next 2 quarters critical**

Industry View: Manish Sabharwal, chairman, TeamLease: Impact can't be modelled. Emotional contagion will have a much longer tail than the virus

MICROORGANISM FACTS FOR KIDS

Negative Impact on Property Market

It definitely came in at the worse time ever. Trade had been crippled eversince the crisis flipped our lives upside down and causing panic fears.

Before the pandemic, house prices in the property market had lost ground and were likely to reach the new highest peak shortly by the end of the year 2020. Then, out of the blue the coronavirus came in and started to take control on every livelihood and along the way, wreaking havoc and leaving a huge dents on country economy to pile up debts and using up all its resources and reserves to salvage the crisis.

Initially, housing prices were holding up steadily. Because of the panic fears in people's mind that going to a showroom or viewing resale house could easily catch the fatal infectious disease, it eventually brought down all the property transaction volumes to a historically low level. It prompted many to stay away from it and to adopt a wait-and-see approach while others are still worrying about job losses, business closures and the spinning of the world economy into recession crisis. Now it is entirely a changed world being taking over by the COVID-19 pandemic that is going to reshape the whole world on how it permanently alters the way we live, work and invest.

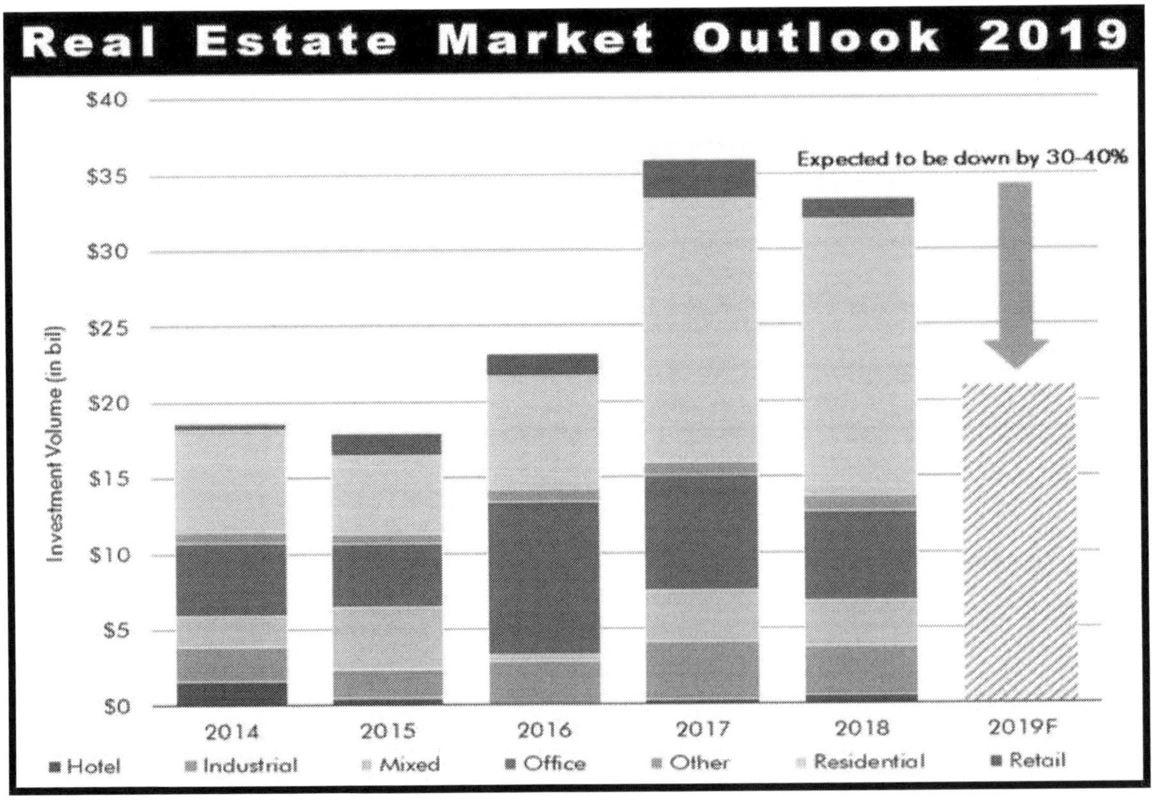

MICROORGANISM FACTS FOR KIDS

The facts of rapid rising rate of unemployment, low consumer confidence level, imminent recession ahead, banking sectors being more prudent and reluctant to lend, imposing immediate changes into bank lending practices, all of these have contributed to a spiral downward trends on the property market outlook.

According to Global Financial Review, the world economy is expected to go into deep recession that can impact the whole property market globally. Economic growth is forecasting that it is unlikely to see any rebound from the impact caused until late of 2021. Interest rates are projected to remain at the current historical lows for the following 3 consecutive years. Meanwhile, government had been using fiscal stimulus packages and community schemes to help the workforce to retain employed and those affected to lessen their livelihood burdens.

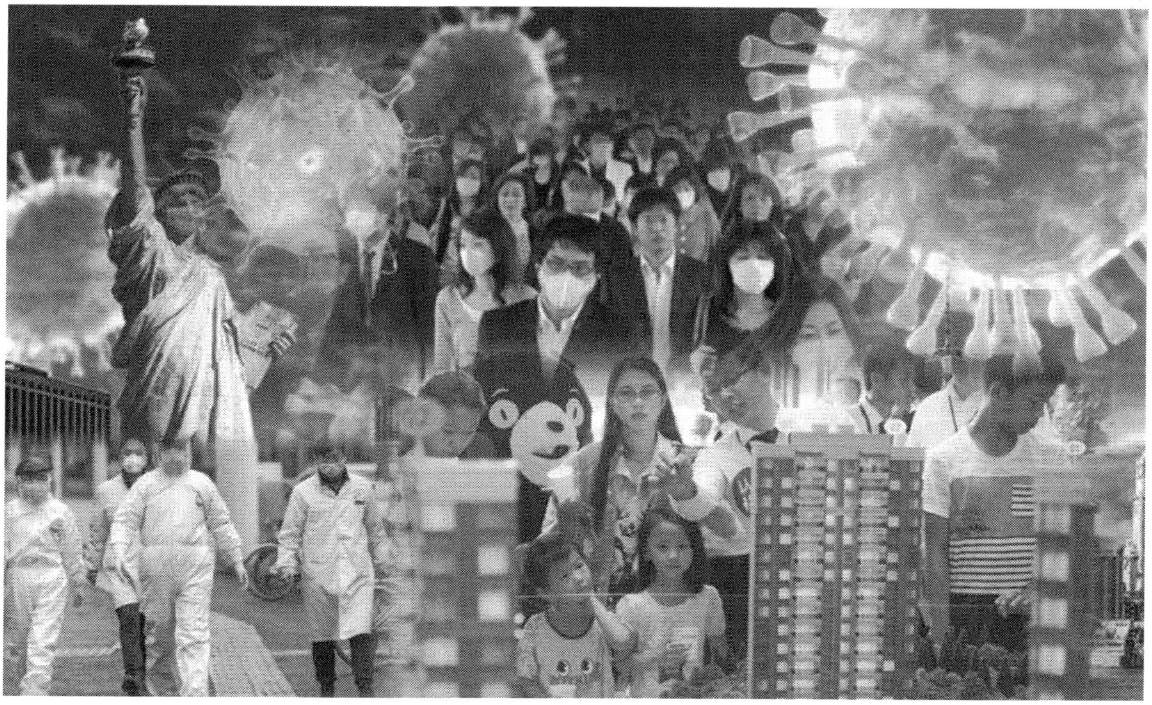

Generally, the impact on the property values is very much dependent on how long it takes to contain the COVID-19 and how severe the harm and damages have been done on the global economies scale.

The worst affected property in the market is usually the more expensive and exclusive ones that will suffer first in line with the stock market crash.

Bank credit lending will be tightened when more local residents suffer from job losses as many businesses are forced to close down due to no consumer spending power in the market.

MICROORGANISM FACTS FOR KIDS

Global Economy Worse Nightmare

If you are trying to sell off your property recently or going to sell it now, you may end up getting only a handful of buyers who may or may not keen to view your property. As time passes, viewers are getting lesser and lesser or even no viewings at all in the sequence months.

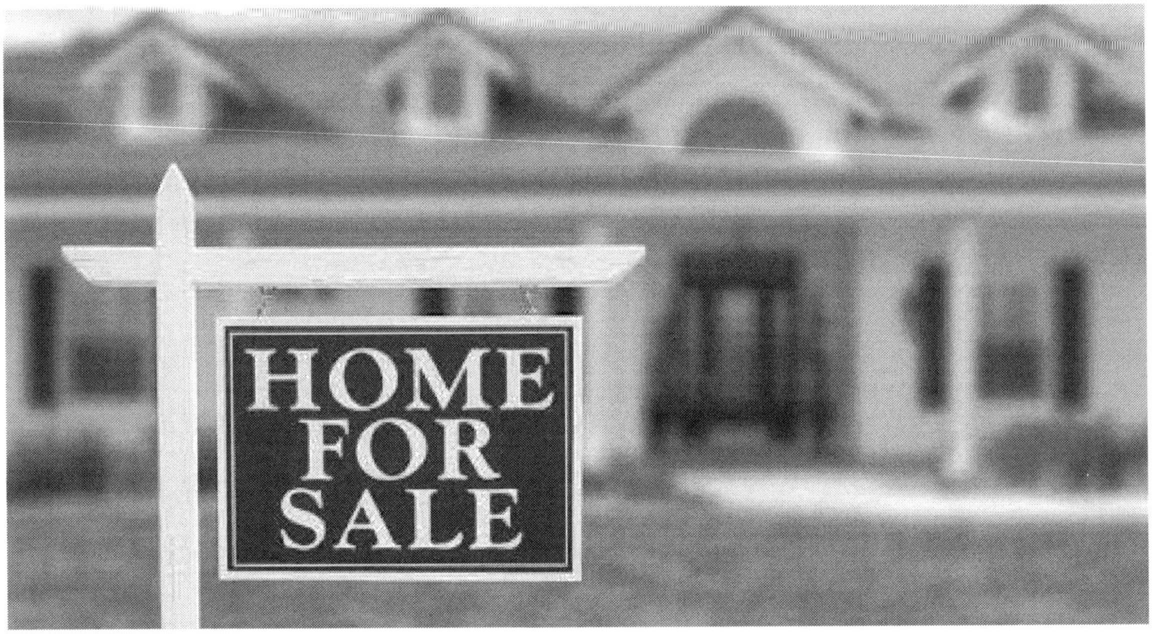

Couple of reasons can be explained why either party, the seller or the buyers, may find it inconvenient to invest their time during which they needed to postpone or cancel their last minute house viewings:

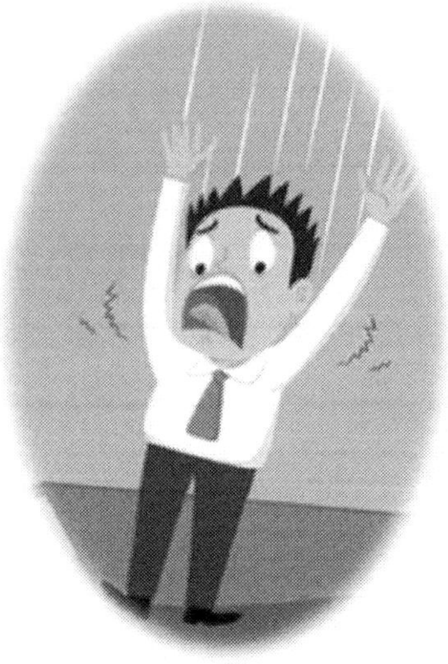

1. Seller is freaking out about the incoming buyers' health conditions who are viewing their house later.
2. Likewise, buyers are also freaking out about entering the seller house. They worry whether any of the seller's family members may have gotten the virus, come in contact with contaminated places or COVID-19 patients, or worse still that any other buyers before them who got the virus infections.
3. When the intended property to view is at or near the virus cluster area, sellers will want to cancel their viewings once they found out that the residence is on that cluster neighbourhood area.

4. Even so, buyers also display uneasiness during house inspection at seller house. They may not like to touch and feel their furniture, go near to their bedroom closets, kitchen and toilet areas etc. to avoid getting infected through contamination surfaces. Every now and then, they will show fears along the inspection process.

   If any of their member is sick and while coughing or sneezing without putting on any face mask, they are definitely going to worry more on themselves that they may get infected too owing to the close proximity social distance apart.

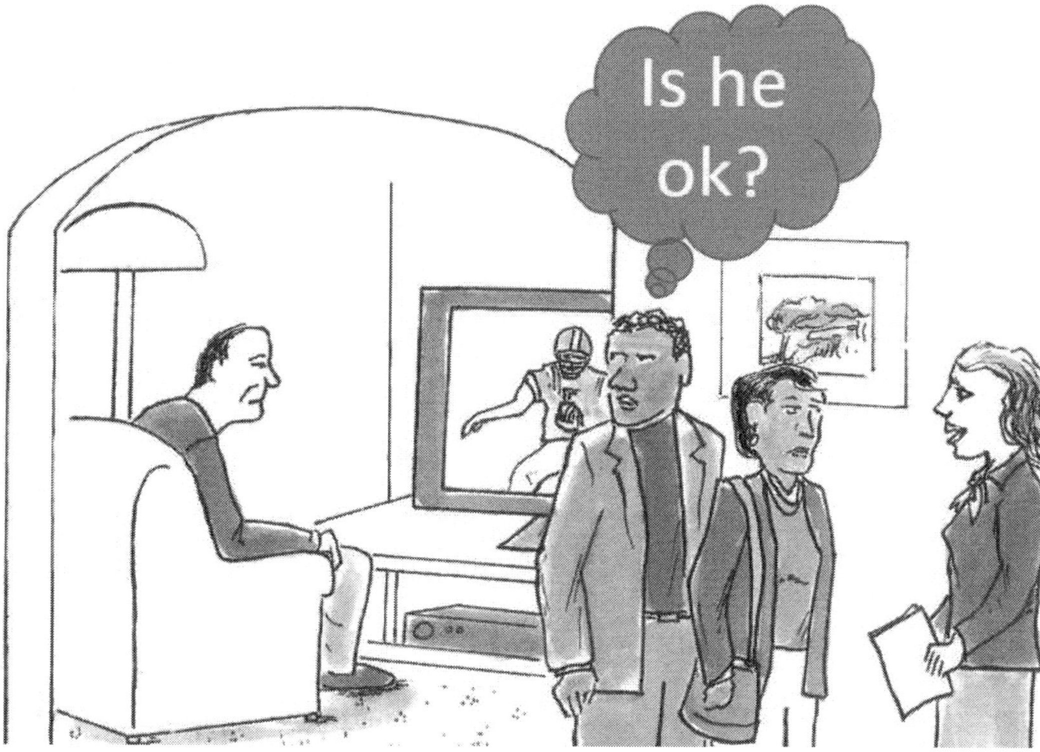

All these worries and concerns that both sellers and buyers have in mind have eventually put on hold on their resale property to view.

Social responsibility is the key to personal hygiene protection.

It still "Better be safe than sorry!"

Unless under unique circumstances where buyers have urgent needs to secure the house and are willing to buy it without conducting any viewing inside.

This may sound a possible arrangement but practically no buyer will take up such arrangement without stepping in and checking the house conditions.

MICROORGANISM FACTS FOR KIDS

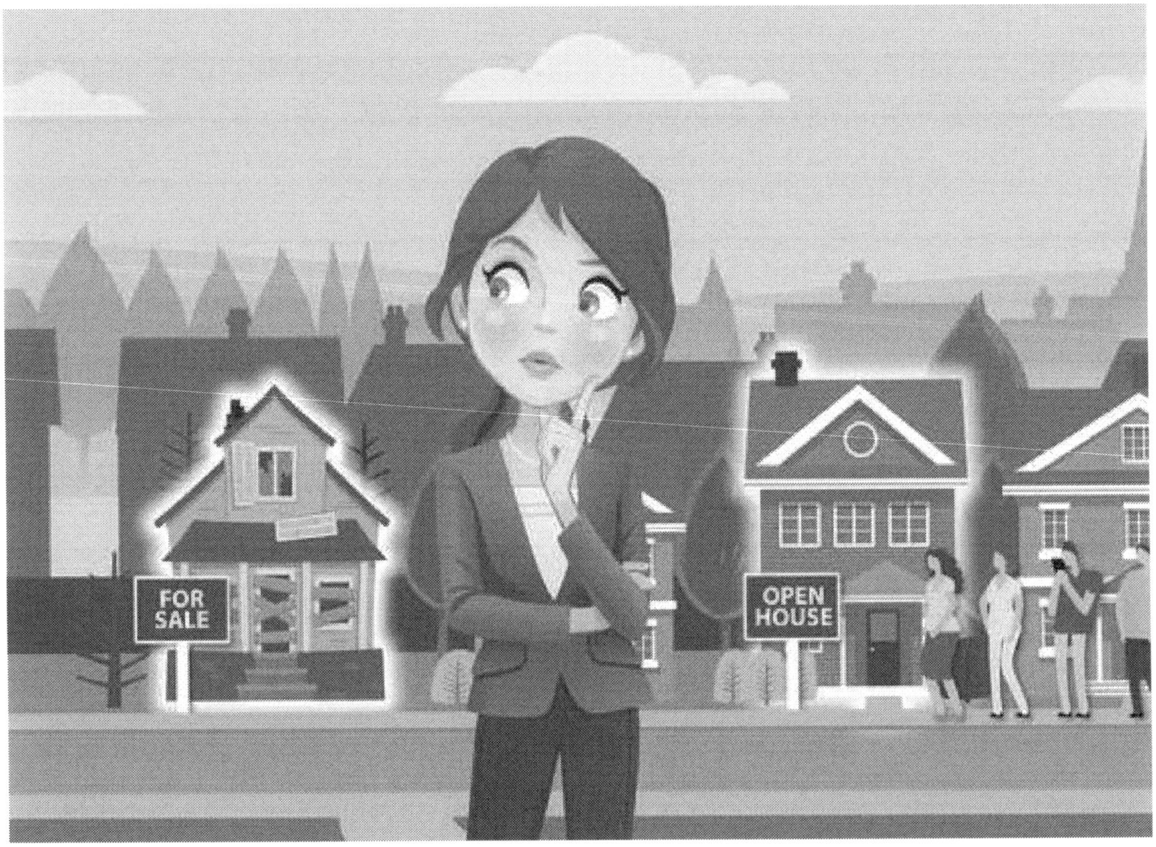

Ok, we finished viewing the house and are pretty close enough to view it from the outside.

Viewing is completed and we can now proceed back to our car. That will be the expected answer you are going to get from the buyers without showing any tell-tale sign that they are keen in this house or not.

Contrary, the resale property market compared to the showflat viewings, resale property carries an even higher risk factors. Unlike showflat, a resale home is actually where people currently lived in.

People and pets may sit and lie on the couch, sleep on the beds, use the toilets frequently, leaving behind any tiny germ particles behind unknowingly.

Houses that are near to the airport and hospital vicinity areas are considering the worst hit with no or lesser viewers expected.

Trying to sell a house is hard. But, trying to sell a house in the middle of a crisis is simply a nightmare, an impossible mission indeed!

Many housing agents can hardly find any seller or buyer at this time.

Property Market Outlook

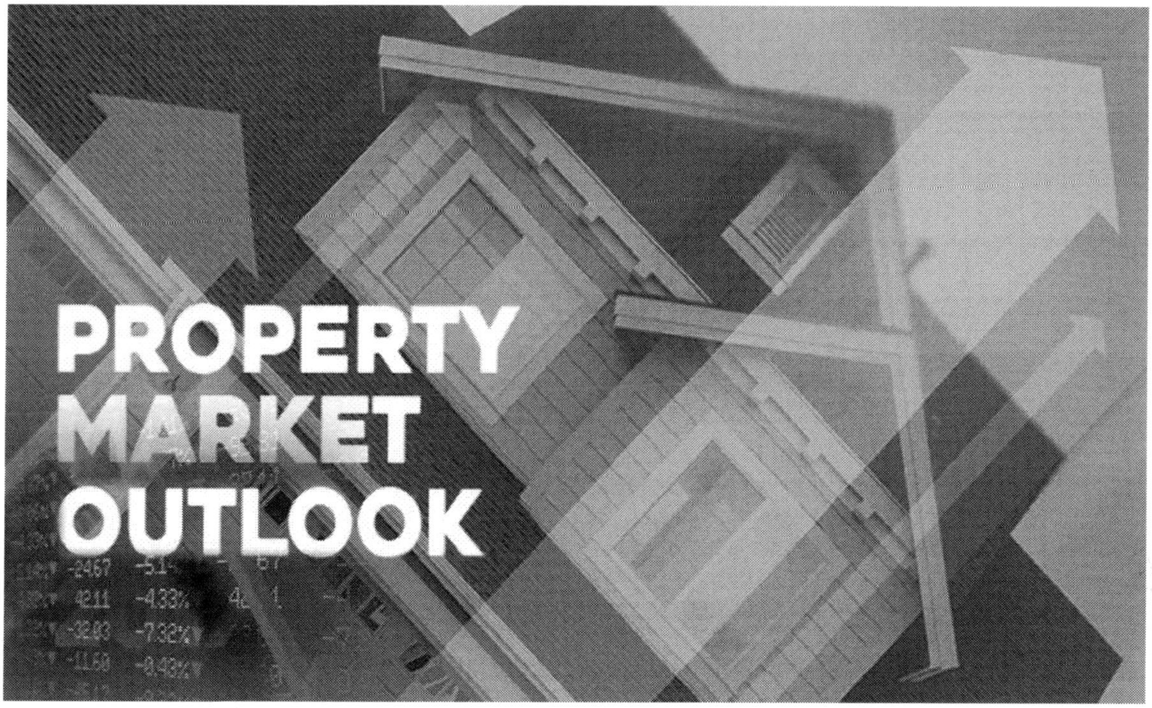

The coronavirus impacts have spiralled the sale transaction volumes, affecting the entire resale market and also the showflat sales.

Commercial and residential property investors alike are adopting a wait-and-see approach while keeping abreast with the world news on the extensive implications of the pandemic's scale of damages incurred on the world economies before plunging their interest back into the real estate market again.

Coupled with the lowest tourism numbers and cutting down flights by airlines, fewer foreign investors are coming in to buy the exclusive properties. Landlords see lesser demand for their properties in-rent advertised on the local papers and social media platforms.

The lockdown measures have totally putting a halt to the country to bar property agents, prospective buyers and valuers from making house visits. Furthermore, any sale closings now may be parked with unforeseen circumstances later on, arising from various practical and financial obstacles that can block its path due to a sudden job loss, confirmed deaths and infections link cases, putting a hold on the property purchase when everybody starts to worry about the coming months as economy is getting worse. Even after the pandemic is over will they still able to secure any good paying jobs that they had held before?

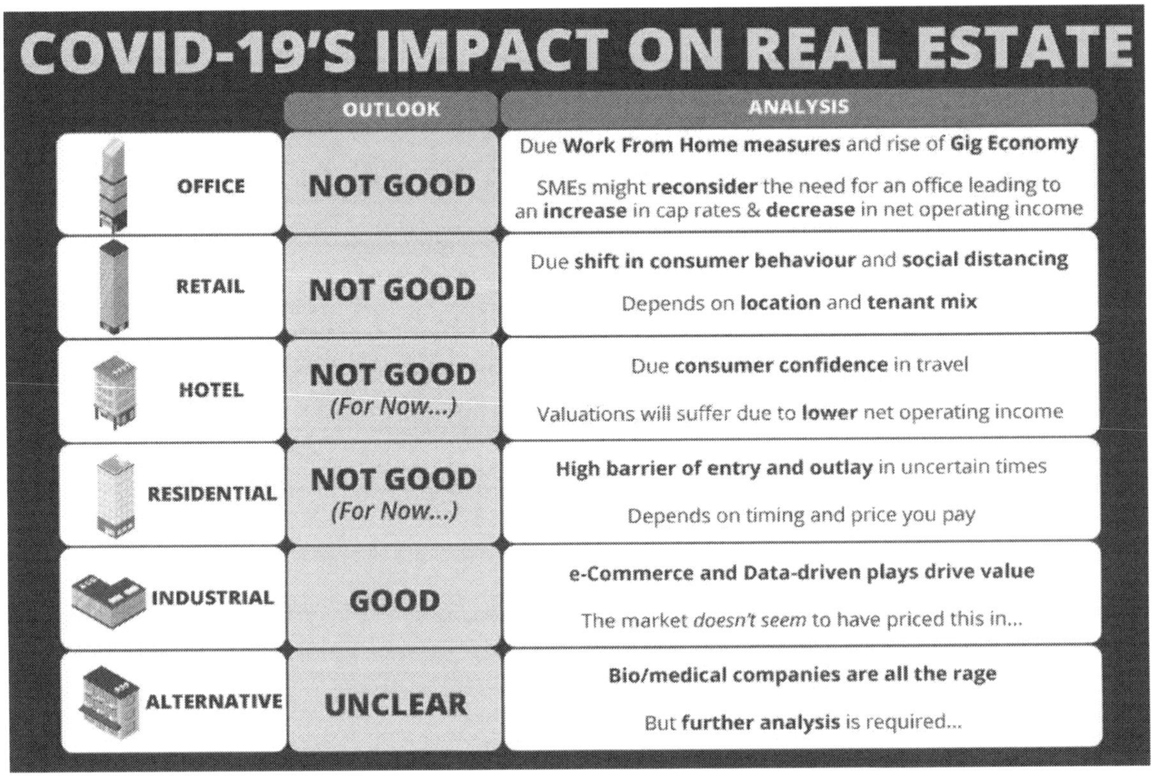

COVID-19'S IMPACT ON REAL ESTATE

	OUTLOOK	ANALYSIS
OFFICE	NOT GOOD	Due **Work From Home measures** and rise of **Gig Economy** SMEs might **reconsider** the need for an office leading to an **increase** in cap rates & **decrease** in net operating income
RETAIL	NOT GOOD	Due **shift in consumer behaviour** and **social distancing** Depends on **location** and **tenant mix**
HOTEL	NOT GOOD *(For Now...)*	Due **consumer confidence** in travel Valuations will suffer due to **lower** net operating income
RESIDENTIAL	NOT GOOD *(For Now...)*	**High barrier of entry and outlay** in uncertain times Depends on timing and price you pay
INDUSTRIAL	GOOD	**e-Commerce and Data-driven plays drive value** The market *doesn't seem* to have priced this in...
ALTERNATIVE	UNCLEAR	**Bio/medical companies are all the rage** But **further analysis** is required...

More shop tenants are also likely to default on their rents or even closing down their businesses entirely due to poor or negligible crowd at all. For those who had already tenanted, they are most likely to offer lower rent than before to keep the tenants, fearing that if getting more frequent delays and more rent defaulters on the rise, they will have difficulty to pay out their bank loan mortgages as more layouts are increasing amid the crisis.

The bad news are that the COVID-19 recession can cause lasting damage to the world economy.

A recession like this is going to see many all types of properties to go under the hammer and start to sell at below market prices.

Many fire sale deals are putting up in the market and bargain hunters will be the ones who happen to be the luckiest buyers to hunt down these undervalued properties as some sellers are so desperate to offload their multiple properties that they had hold previously.

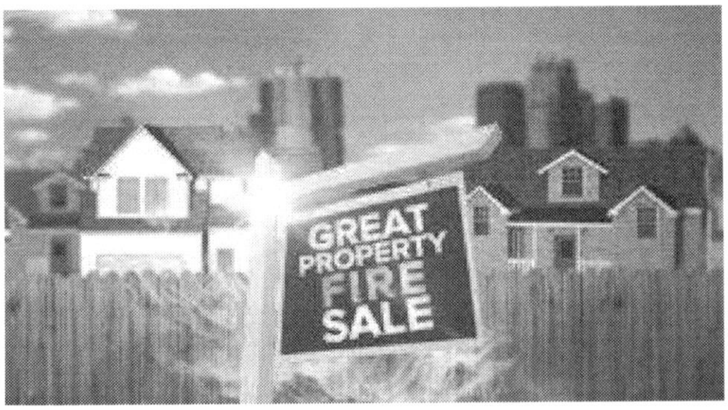

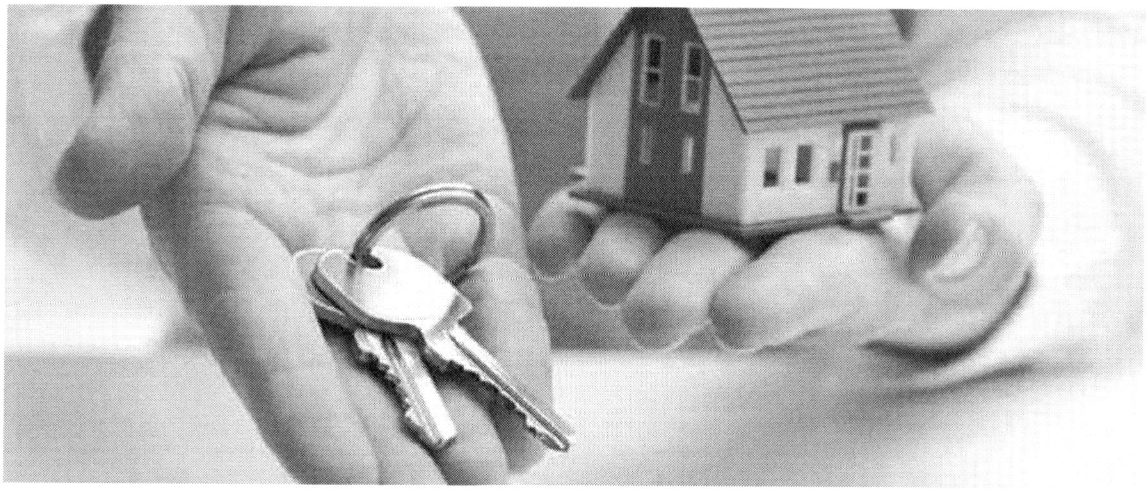

Generally, the overall scenario in the showrooms sales of new launch property, developers are giving out deep discounts and delay progressive instalments for the purchase of their new launch property to induce buyers to seal the purchase agreement as quick as possible before the market turns even worse.

The discounts and the delay progressive payments make the sale transaction more appealing and affordable pricing to these prospective buyers who are planning to purchase their private dream home.

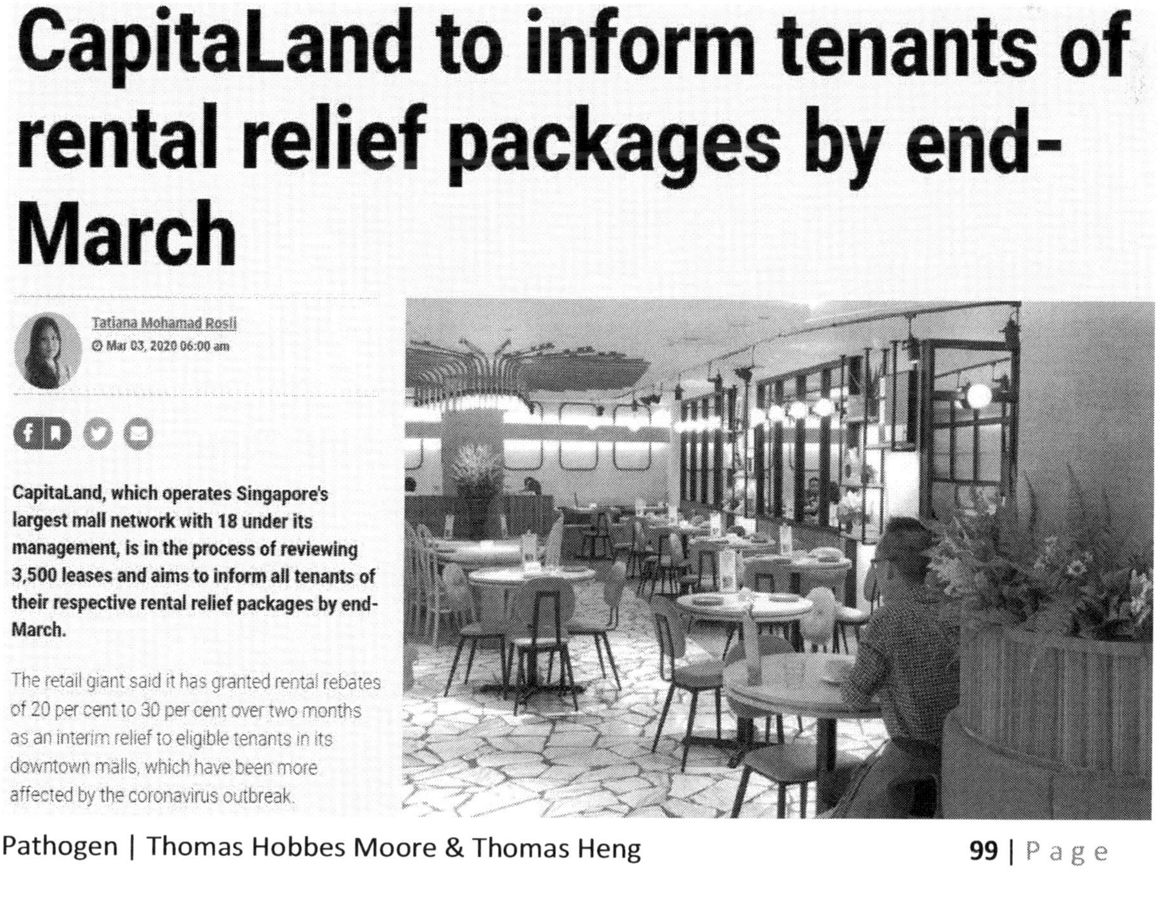

CapitaLand to inform tenants of rental relief packages by end-March

Tatiana Mohamad Rosli
Mar 03, 2020 06:00 am

CapitaLand, which operates Singapore's largest mall network with 18 under its management, is in the process of reviewing 3,500 leases and aims to inform all tenants of their respective rental relief packages by end-March.

The retail giant said it has granted rental rebates of 20 per cent to 30 per cent over two months as an interim relief to eligible tenants in its downtown malls, which have been more affected by the coronavirus outbreak.

The panic fears put an emergency brakes on the real estate stocks amidst market sell-off

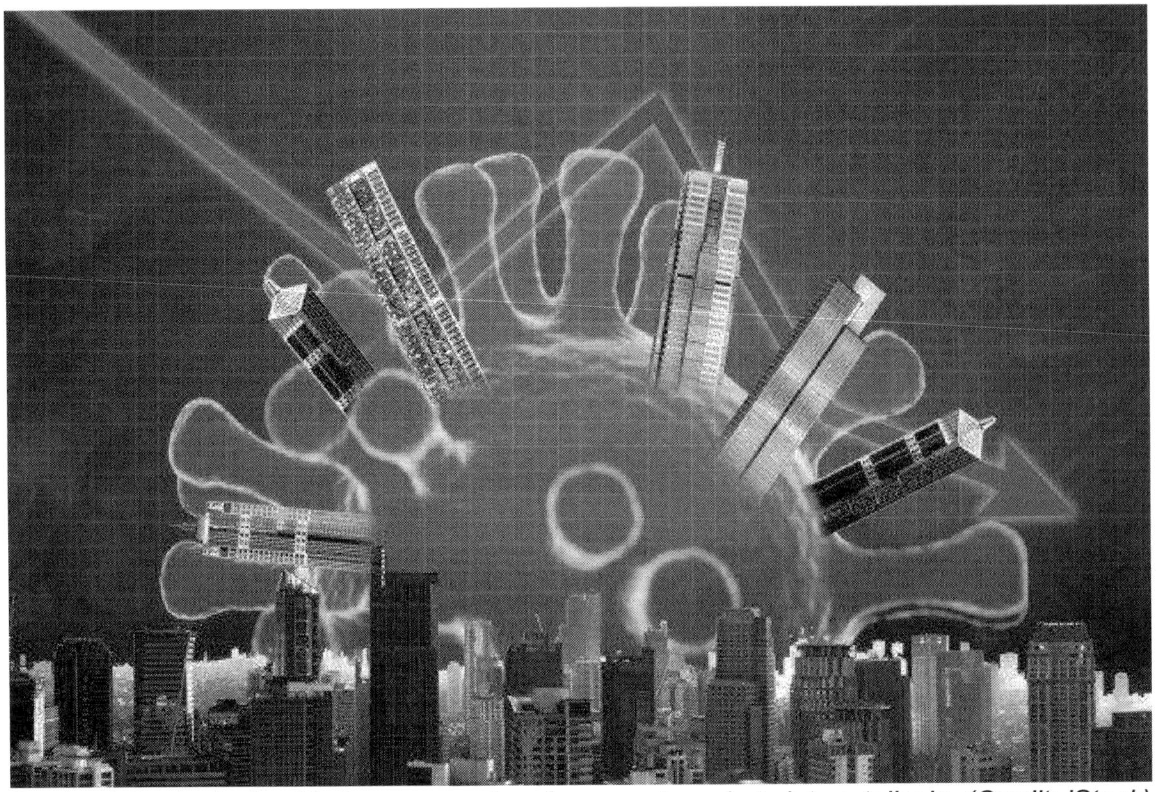

Real estate stocks tumbled as coronavirus fears sent markets into a tailspin. (Credit: iStock)

Real estate in hotels and retail industry have been becoming the worst stock performers as comparing to the other sectors in the industry.

They are seen to be the causalities hardest hit in this miserable year 2020 on REITs, real estate investment trusts, where its losses are accumulating and accelerating over time.

Their stock shares plummet amid the panic fears and lead many shares selloff before the end of the day.

REITs' fundamentals and earnings all spiralling down like a tsunami as compared to other equity stock performances.

Property mortgage rates went into a spiral spin downward as investors are fleeing to other safe havens stocks while pushing the housing mortgage rates to a near historical lows.

The interest rates are low and can go down further too. The prevailing low interest rate is attractively a pull factor to own a home easier now either as an owner occupier or a property investor who are cash rich.

Microorganism Facts For Kids

Coronavirus Crisis Respond Calls with Technology

AI Robotics Community

In the face of the pandemic, advanced countries like Japan, China and Singapore have been turning to AI robotics to adopt surveillance technologies in an action call for the robotics community to coronavirus fears of the human transmission.

Develop by the Chinese Academy of Sciences, these robots are deployed in places like hospitals to remotely help nurses to collect swabs from patient after swab testing, despatch medicines, deliver food and documents to the isolation room doorstep where patients stay in during their self-isolating period.

The intelligent robots can play a vital role in self-managing itself to enter the lift, knock on the patient room and call the patient out to open the door. Robotics community provides robotics challenges and deploying their use in the areas where mission is impossible to reach for disasters, logistics, drones and infectious diseases. For examples in research areas of interest in:

1. Surgical robotics
2. Rehabilitation and assistive robots
3. Hospital and laboratory automation process

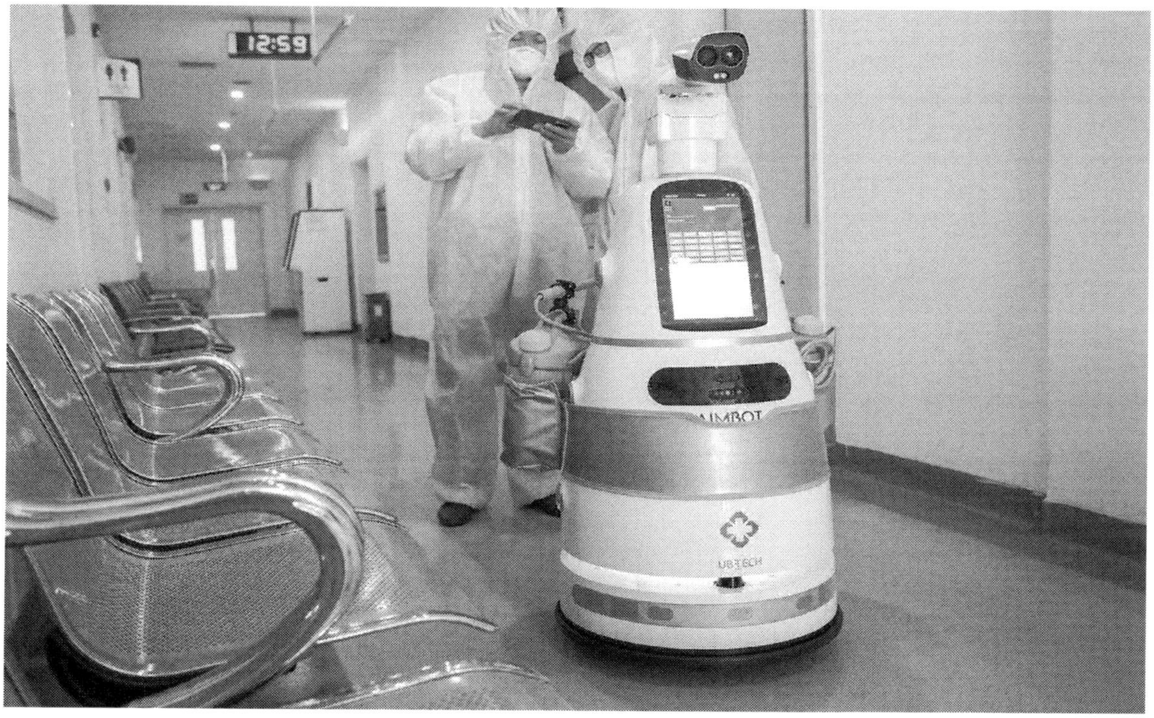

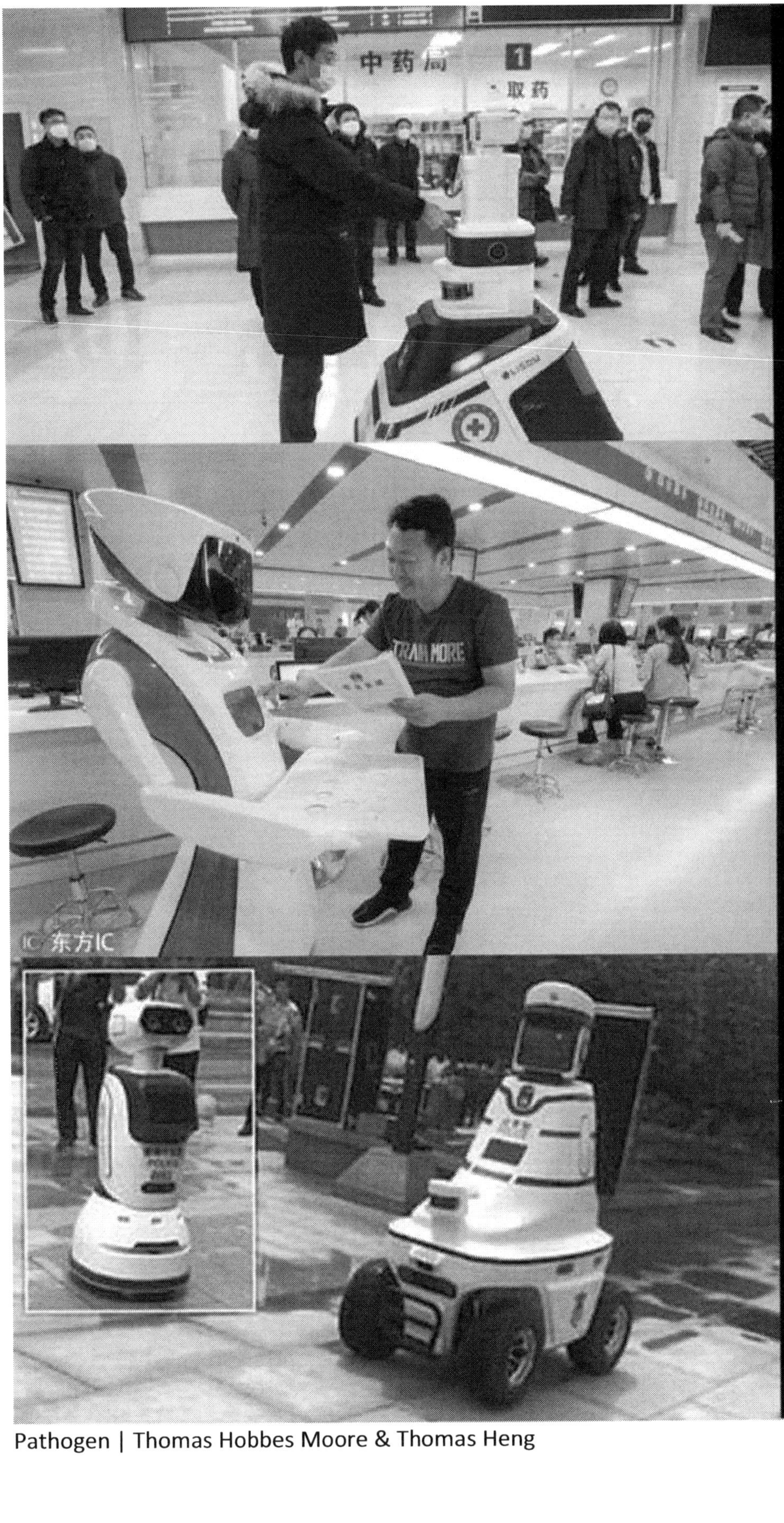

Robotics Commuity

MICROORGANISM FACTS FOR KIDS

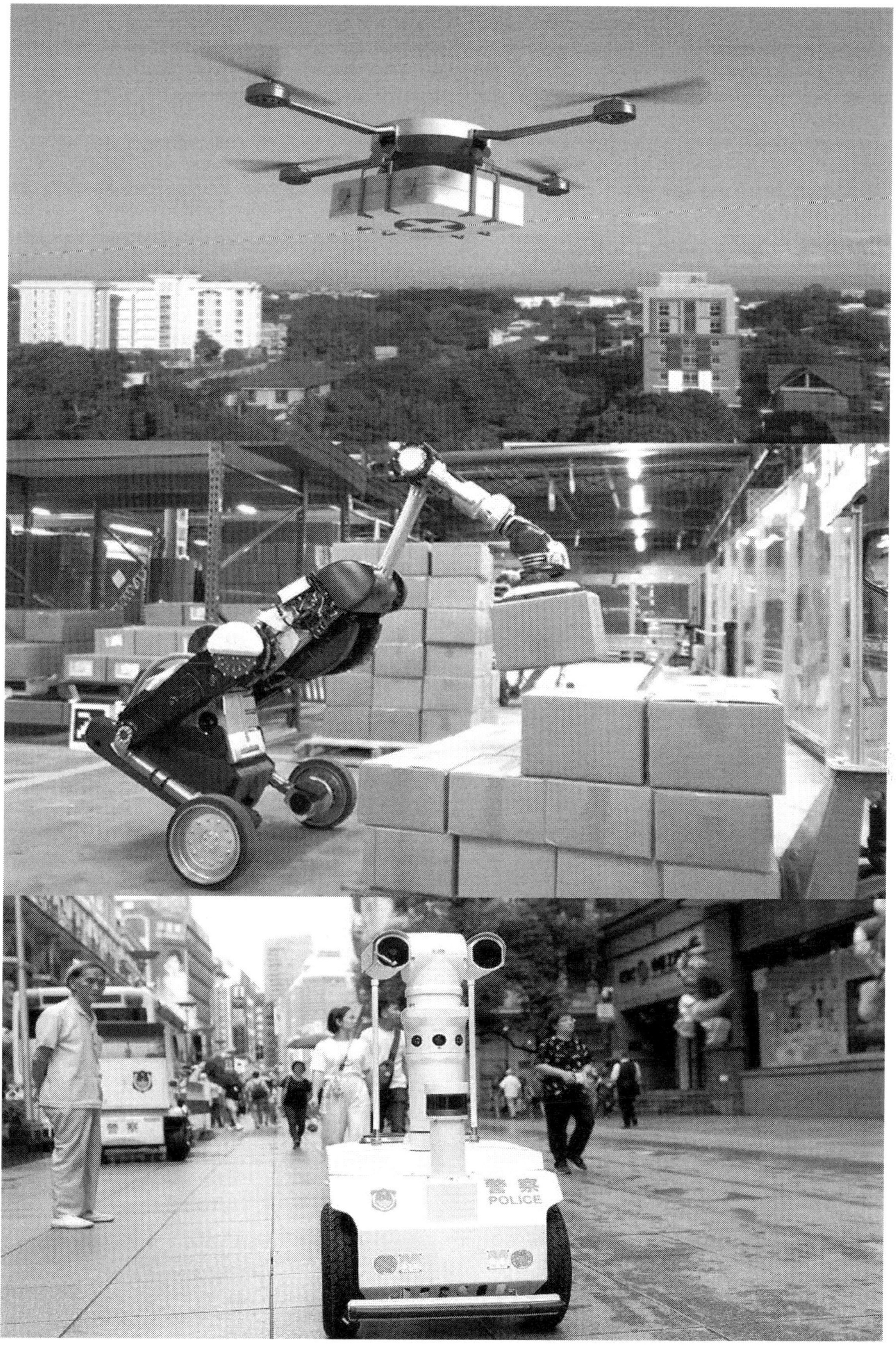

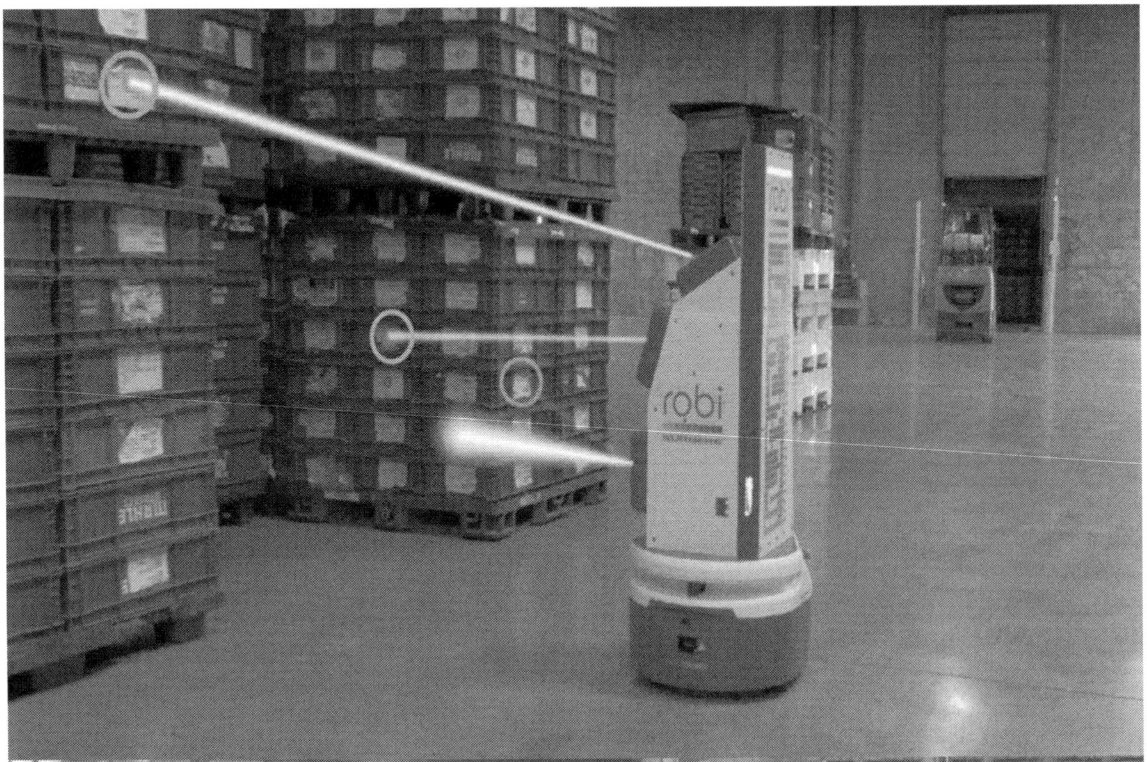
robi

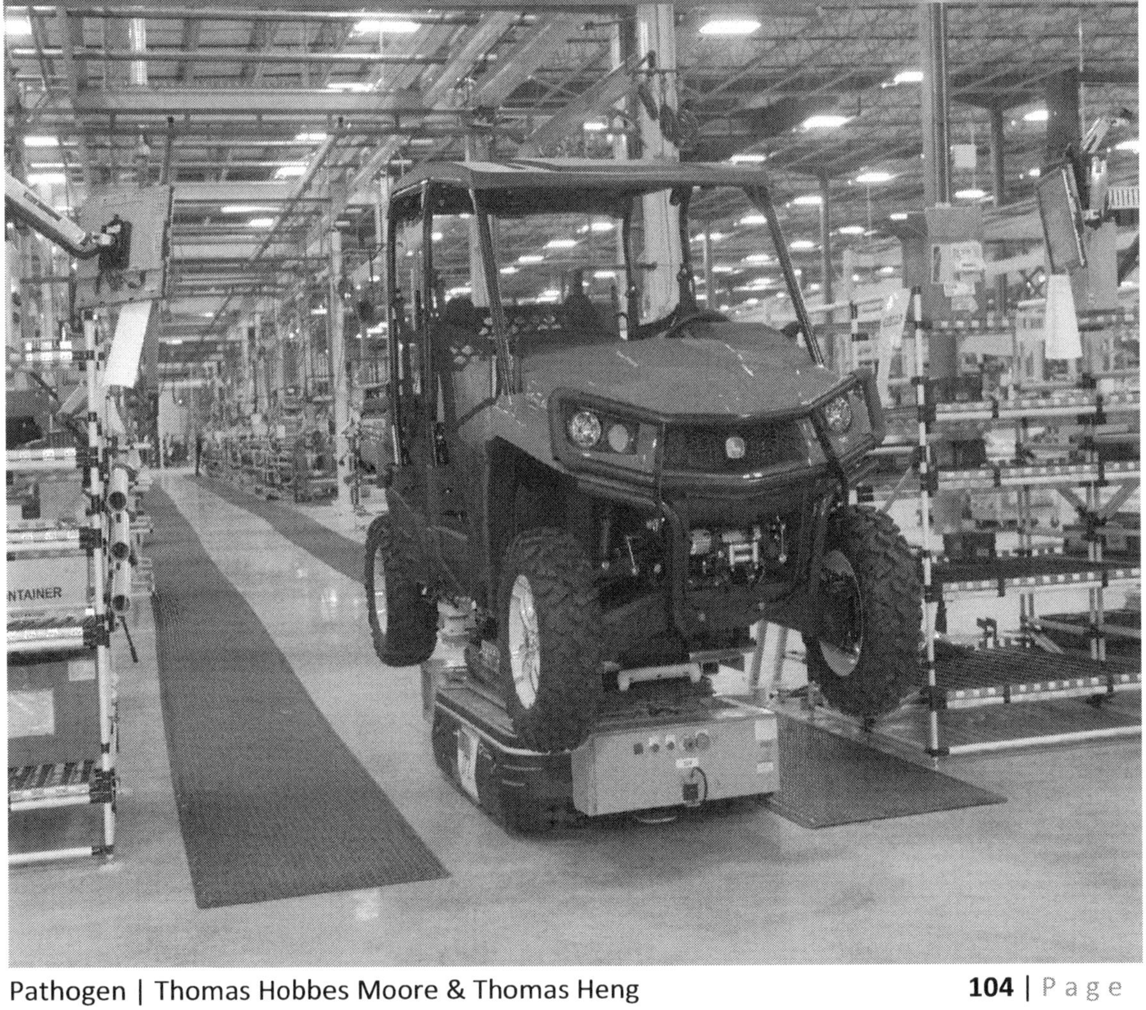

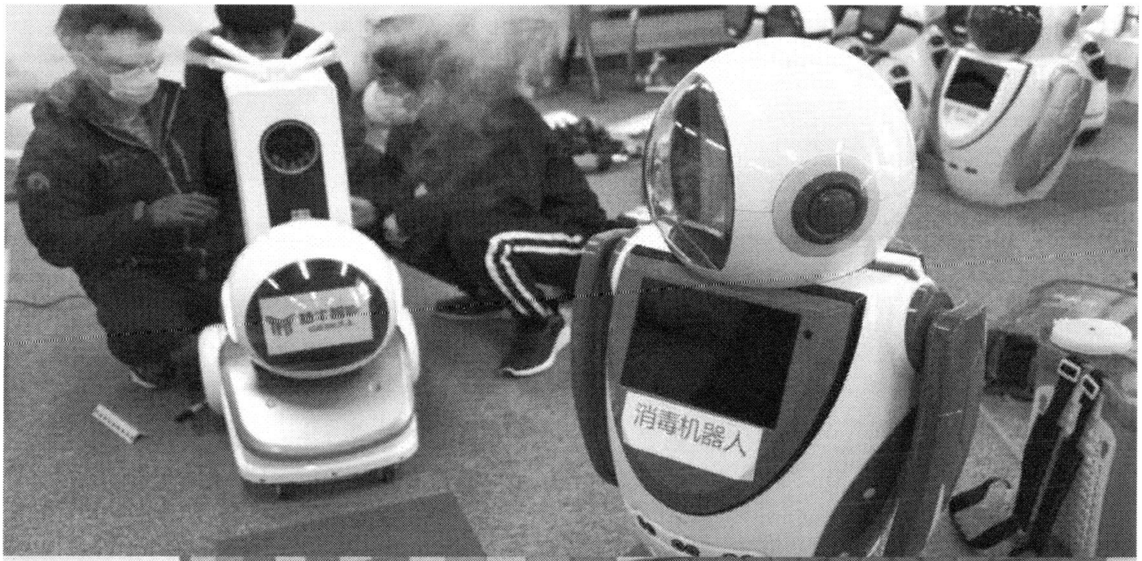
消毒机器人

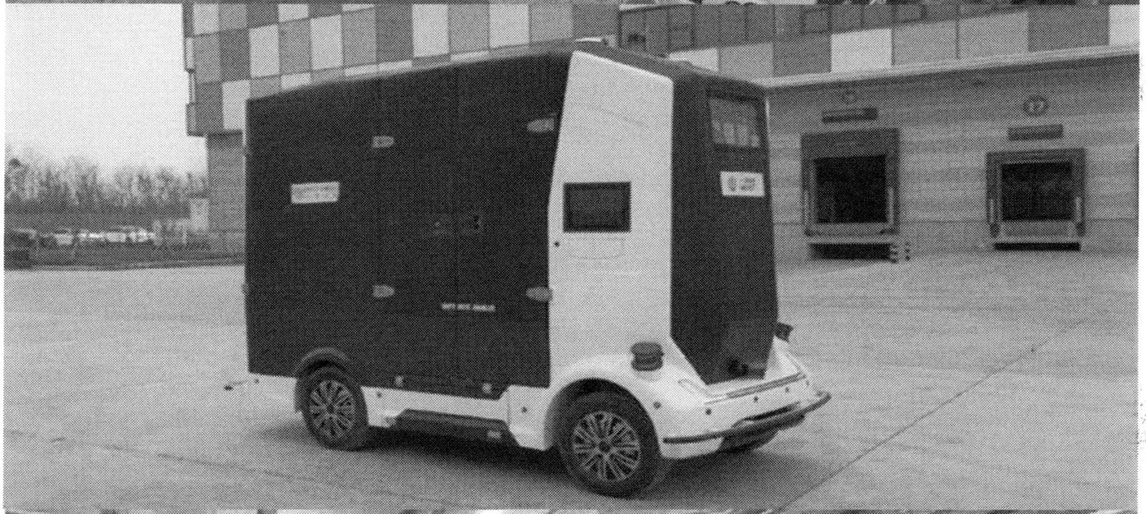

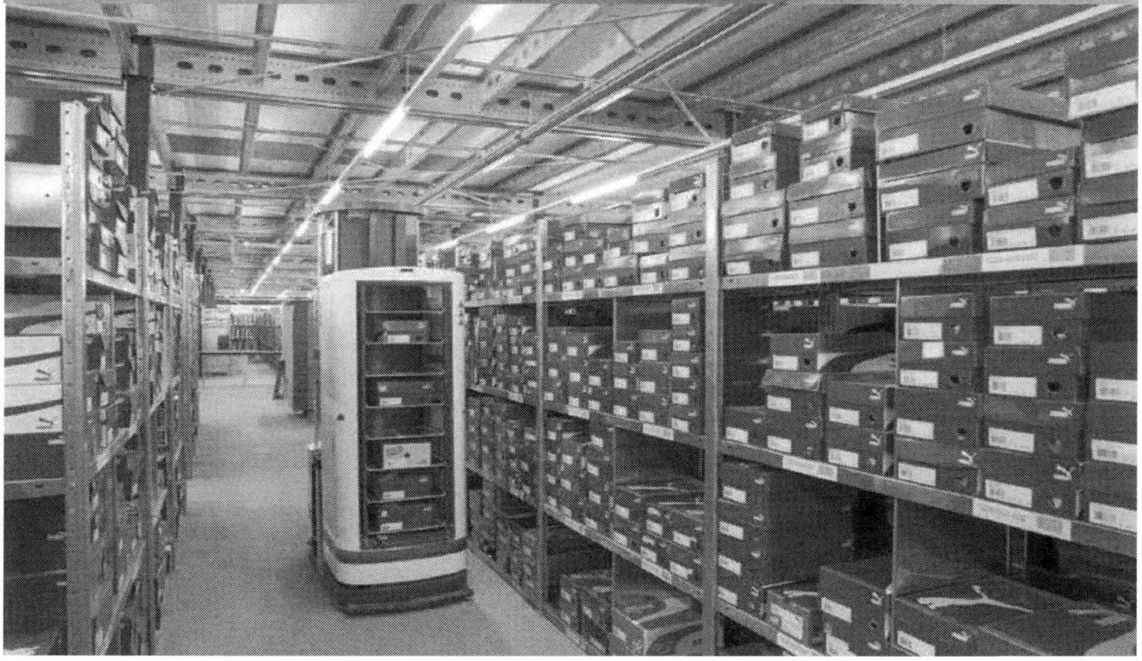

Adopting Surveillance Technologies

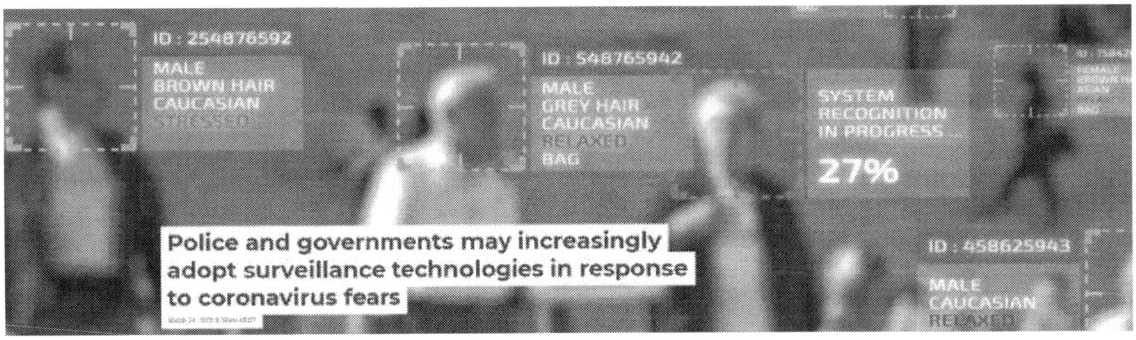

Welcome to the futuristic world of technology.

Surveillance technologies concept is on the pipeline. Federal government is planning to get police forces to adopt Clearview AI, Artificial Intelligent, facial recognition to track its people movement and whereabouts in the country and increasingly relying on it to manage people for data and analysis collection.

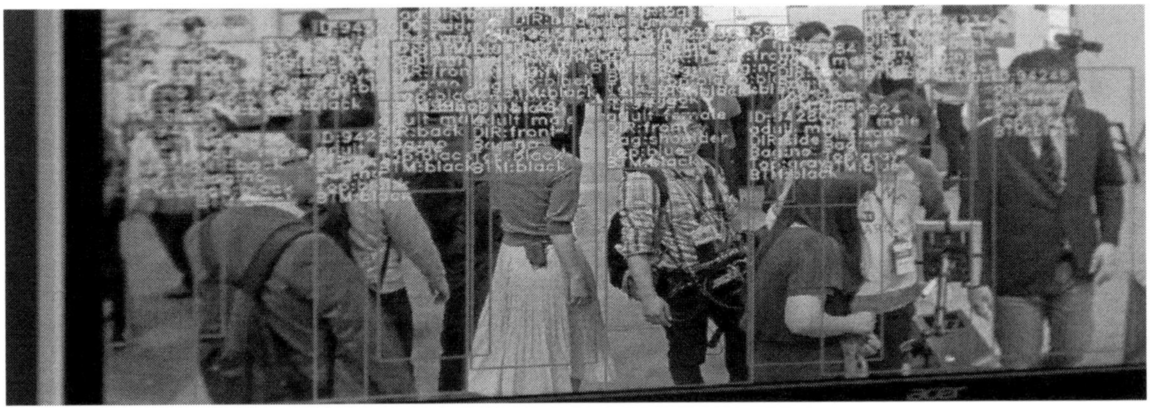

Deploying the surveillance technologies in this pandemic situation help to track symptomatic and asymptomatic carriers in the country to gather all the multimodal information and collate it centrally and systematizing on the active catalog system.

Up-to-date information can interlink and transferred via high speed link to Johns Hopkins University for scientists, infectious experts and government agency to have obtain information at a much shorter and faster access rate time for their studies, investigation and detail analysis purposes.

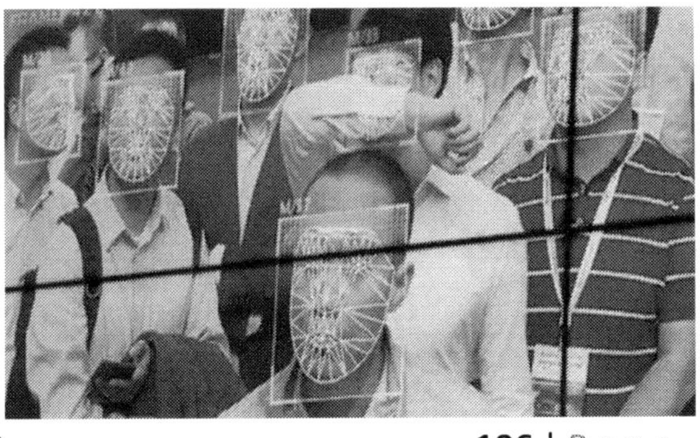

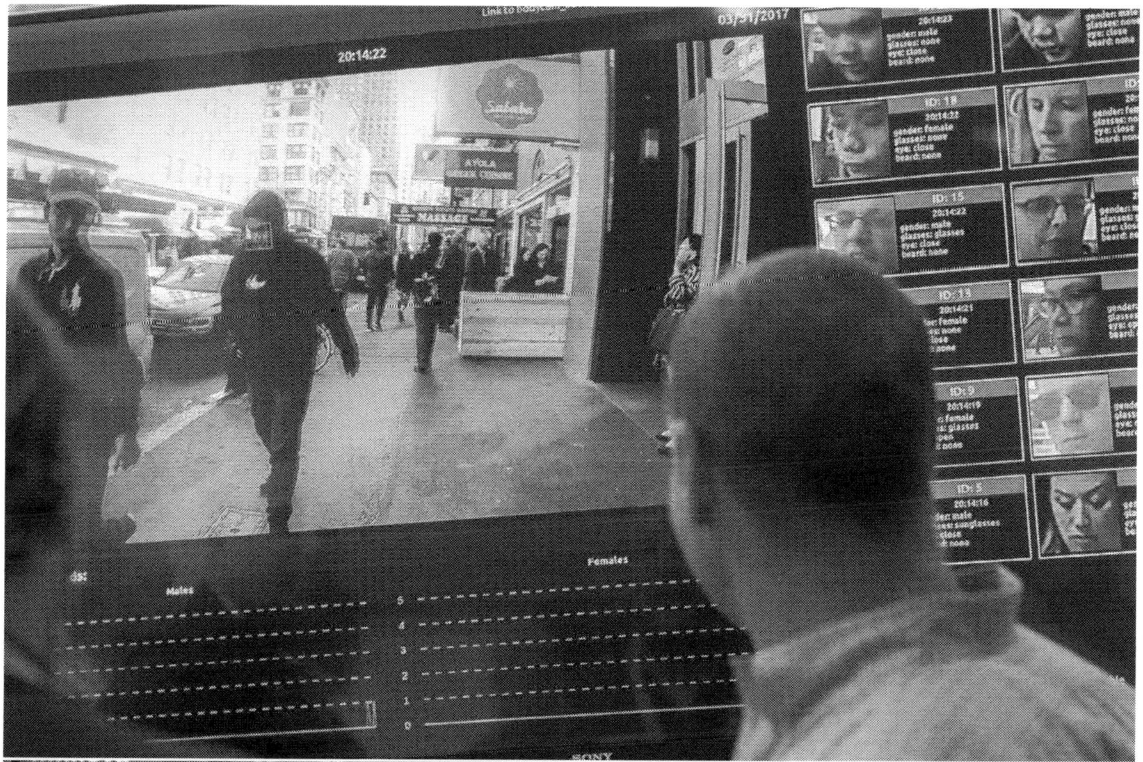

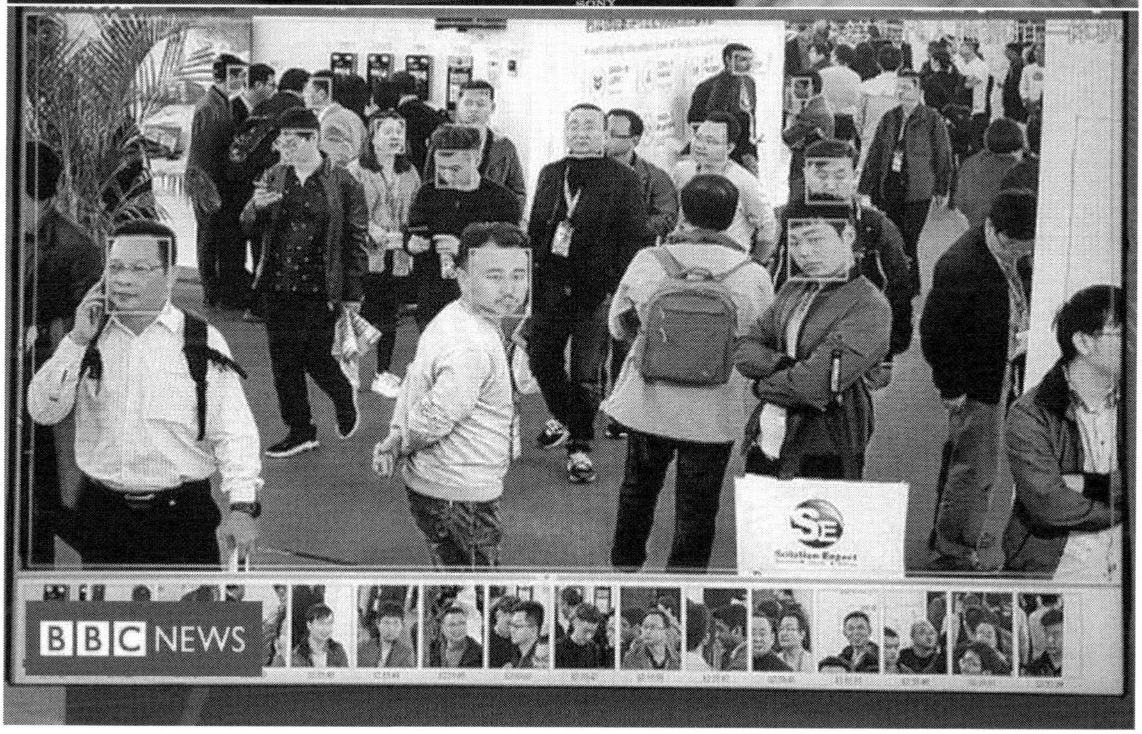

The main drawback for implementing such surveillance technology is one can expect loss of personal data privacy to be breached since the system can exploit these information at will and does its matching algorithms and extracting individual and other photos of his across multiple social media platforms at the split of a second.

This leads to a question of security breaches on personal privacy data carrying out on both accidental and intentional causes.

Because of these reasons, policing of personal data integrity and its privacy need to be thoroughly debated before reaching the conclusive verdict of deploying the use of surveillance technology by police agencies in the first place.

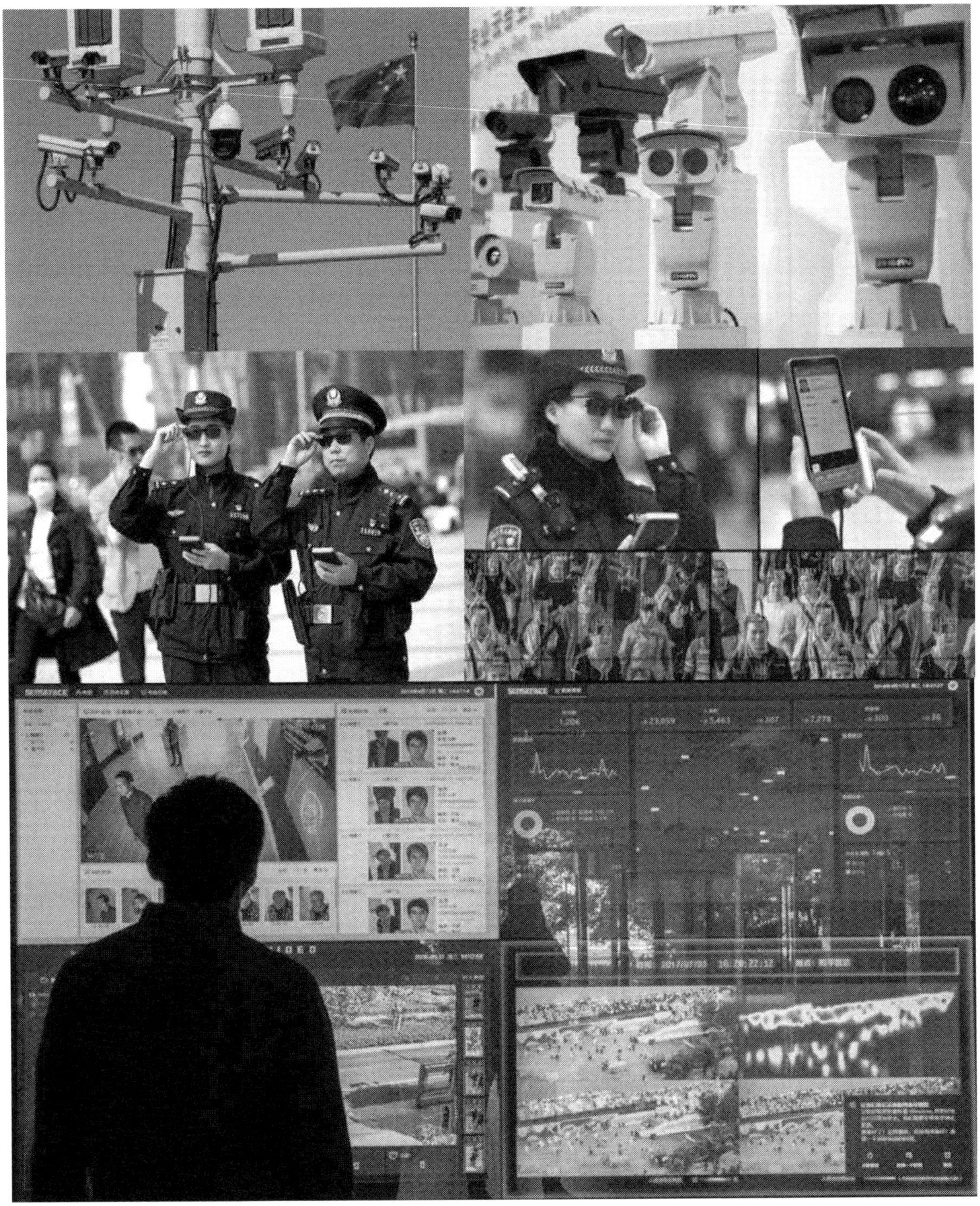

MICROORGANISM FACTS FOR KIDS

Contact-Tracing Apk (TraceTogether): Singapore

Singapore government releases the **TraceTogether** apk, an open-sourced code's contact-tracing app developed by the Government Technology Agency (GovTech). It is freely available. TraceTogether uses Bluetooth technology to find out who have come in contact with you, but does not store the location where the places you had been to.

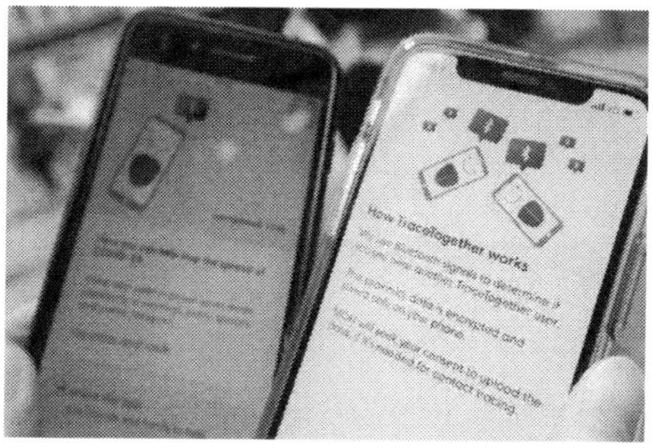

To date, more than 700,000 downloads worldwide had been installed on individual smartphones via the Android Google PlayStore or Apple IOS AppStore. The apk will be deactivated once the pandemic is over.

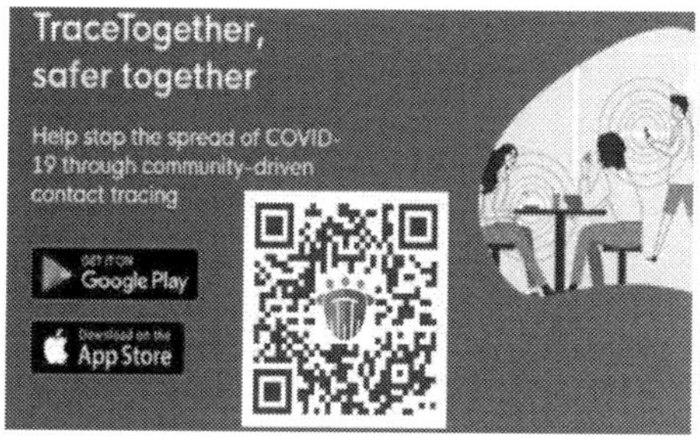
TraceTogether,
safer together
Help stop the spread of COVID-19 through community-driven contact tracing
Google Play
App Store

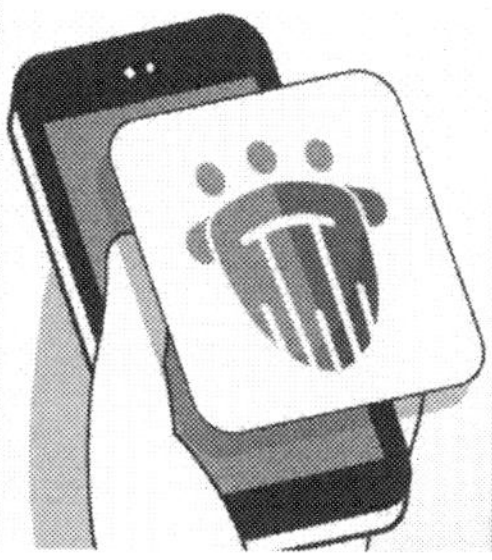

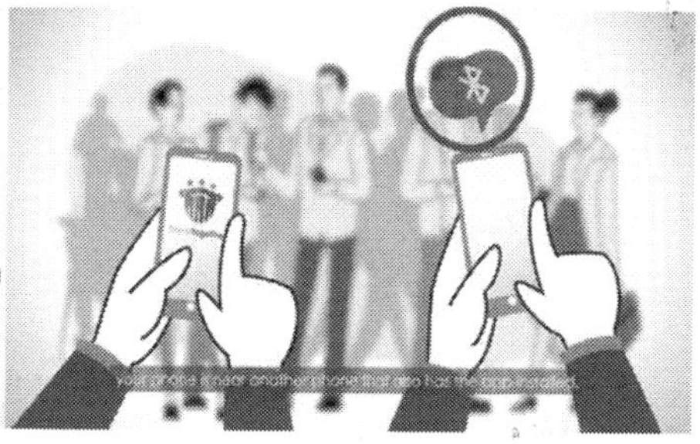

For TraceTogether app to work, the Bluetooth function setting on the smartphone needs to turn on first. The Bluetooth signal is a must and it will automatically help the **contact tracers** to quickly call the victim once the person is in close proximity range of 2m (6 feet) from the COVID-19 patient. All encrypted Bluetooth proximity data are stored inside the individual smartphone. Moreover, this app comes in useful and handy for people who tend to forget or cannot remember whom they are in near contact with when out on their own.

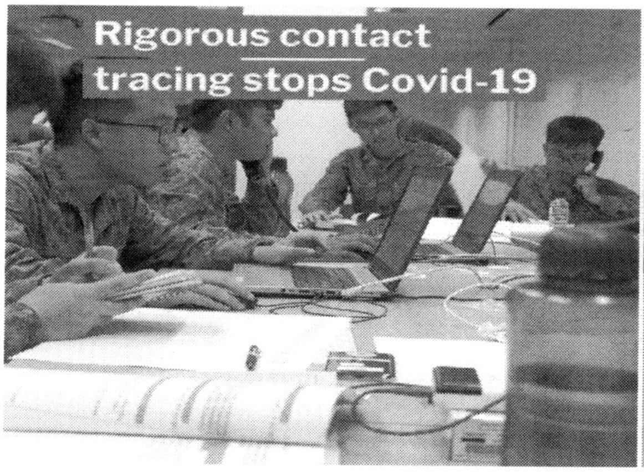
Rigorous contact
tracing stops Covid-19

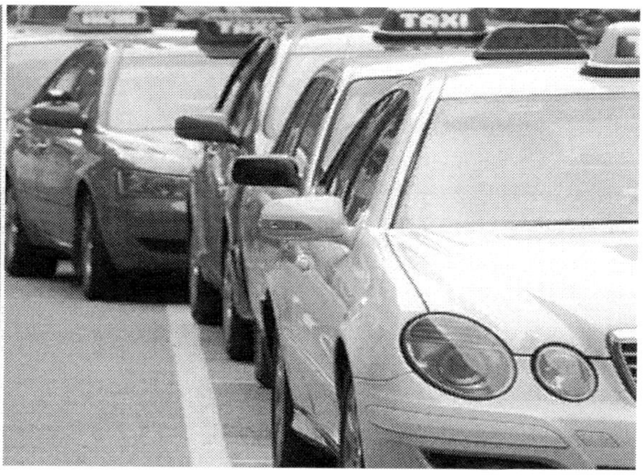
TAXI

MICROORGANISM FACTS FOR KIDS

Those COVID-19 patient is given a verification code by the official contact tracers. If the code on that patient authenticates and matches with the contact-tracing smartphone app, it will transmit a data signal to the contract tracer center.

The contact tracers from the Health Ministry can make quick response and adopt appropriate approach. They will make a call to inform the person that he is within a close range with the infected patient.

By this method of tapping on digital broadband technology via the tracing apps, earlier identification and prevention of potential cases from happening are possible to contain and prevent further spread of the virus to elsewhere.

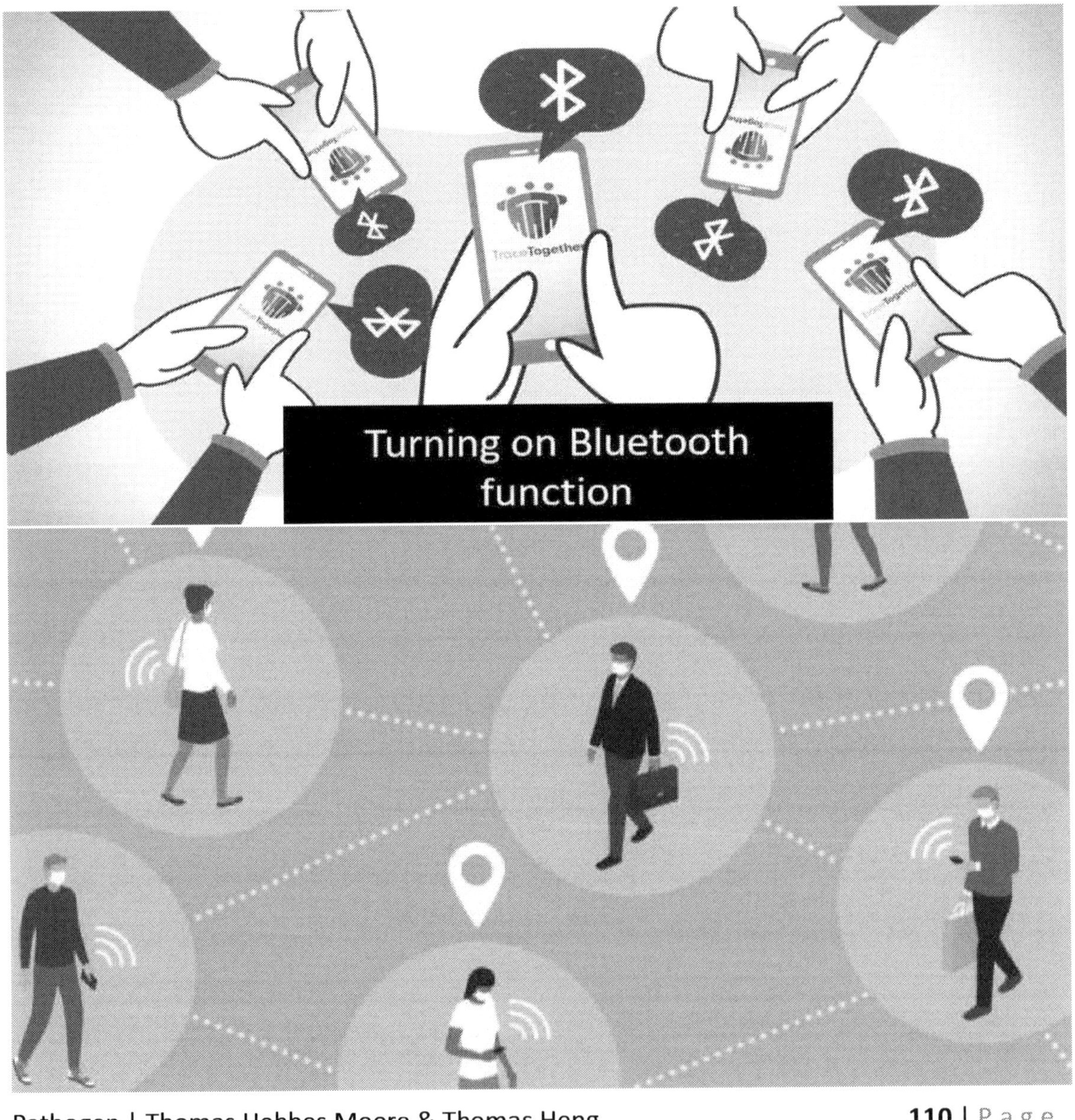

Symptom-Monitoring Apk (COVIDradar): UK

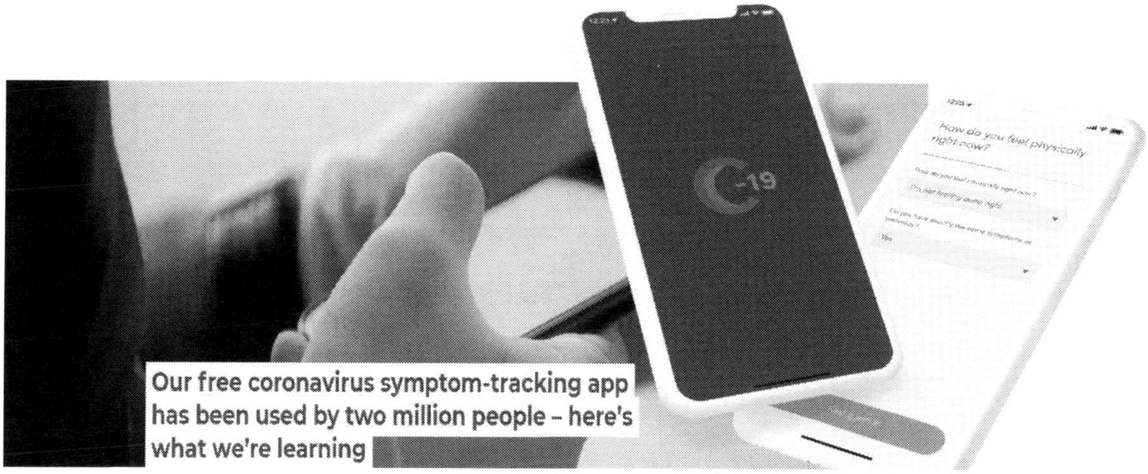

UK releases **COVIDradar** app, a simple symptom-monitoring app developed by the health data science company ZOE, made freely available for downloads via Google PlayStore and Apple IOS Store. Soon this app is also made available to the U.S. region. To date nearly 2 million downloads had been installed in UK on every smartphone.

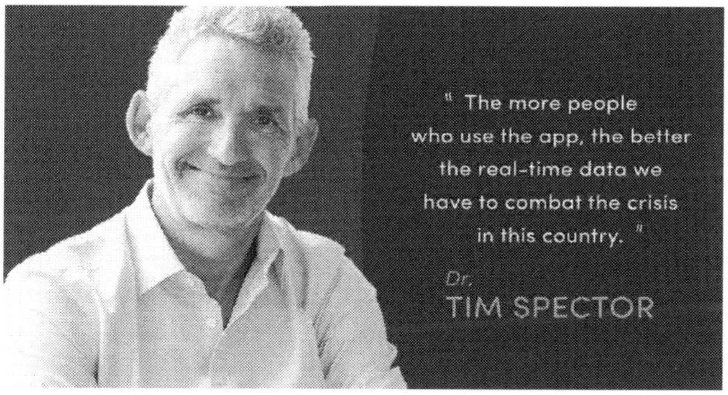
" The more people who use the app, the better the real-time data we have to combat the crisis in this country. "
Dr.
TIM SPECTOR

It gathers and collates information from volunteers who submit their daily health status through the apps, including individual's medical history of microbiome and lifestyle, all being captured into the centralised system.

The data collated offers a significant help in identifying who need to go for the coronavirus swab test based on their current and past coronavirus infection history record.

From the information collated, the appearance of any new COVID infection cases on a population-wide scale can be monitored. It allows policymakers, academic researchers and scientists to study the patterns of these virus symptoms and to find out which group of people is at the highest health risk factor to the virus infection, the rate of its means of spread and to quickly identify and contain the virus clustering areas at the tip of the data. In addition, it aid them to distribute equally on country's resources allocation more efficiently and policy makers can roll out timely and effective policy measures accordingly.

Health QR Colour Codes: China

Alibaba and Tencent companies develop a health QR code apps.

The Chinese government have mandatory instructed their authorities on their respective provinces to roll out these health code app from the **WeChat and Alipay** platforms.

All localities must register and have the app installed on their smartphone to track suspected virus infection cases that the person may have come in contact with any of the coronavirus patient. There are 3 different kinds of colour coding of green, yellow and red that tied to their ID number, showing their current travelling patterns and vital health history records.

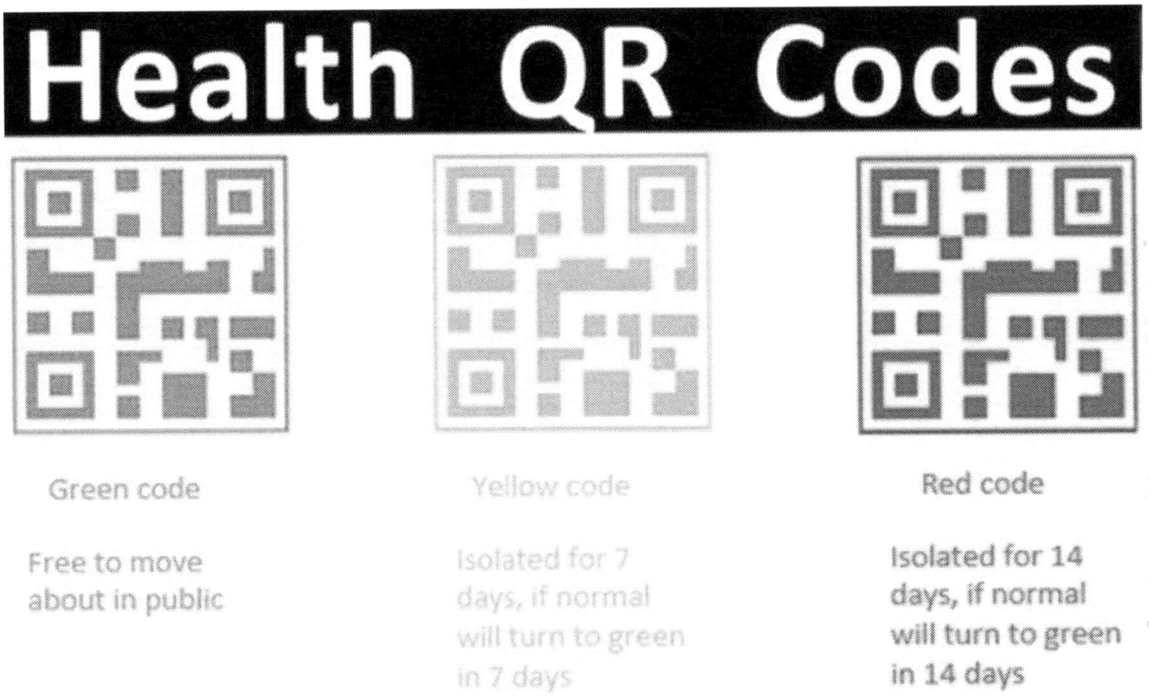

Immuni App: Italy

Develop by Milan-based technology start-up company, Bending Spoons, for the coronavirus location-tracing in the European community.

Applying Bluetooth technology to trace coronavirus patient in close proximity range and sent an automatic alert on the user smartphone.

The Immuni apps are used on voluntarily basis governed under Italy's data privacy policy.

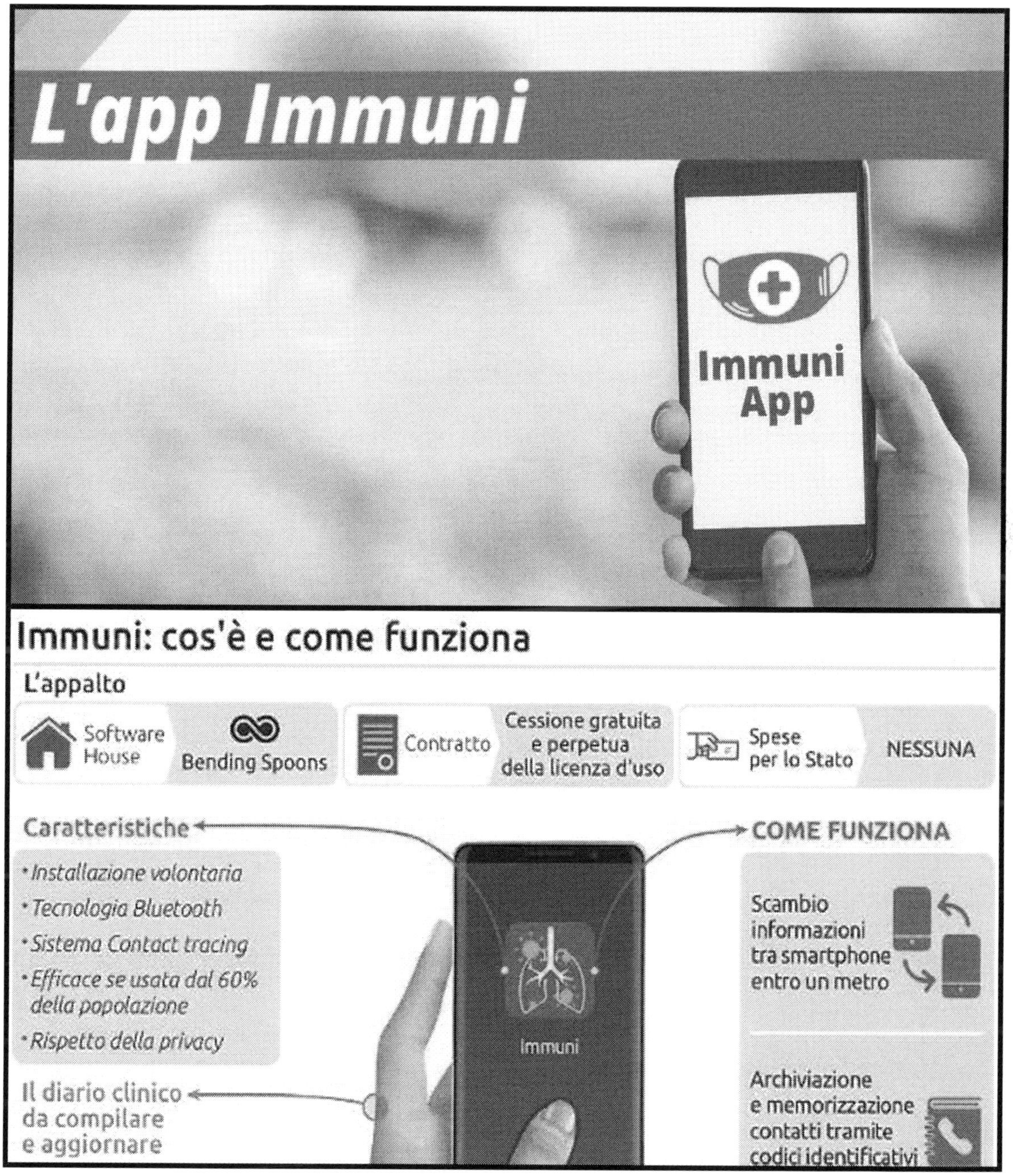
L'app Immuni
Immuni App
Immuni: cos'è e come funziona
L'appalto
Software House
Bending Spoons
Contratto
Cessione gratuita e perpetua della licenza d'uso
Spese per lo Stato
NESSUNA
Caratteristiche
•Installazione volontaria
•Tecnologia Bluetooth
•Sistema Contact tracing
•Efficace se usata dal 60% della popolazione
•Rispetto della privacy
Il diario clinico da compilare e aggiornare
Immuni
COME FUNZIONA
Scambio informazioni tra smartphone entro un metro
Archiviazione e memorizzazione contatti tramite codici identificativi

COVIDSafe Coronavirus Tracking app: Australia

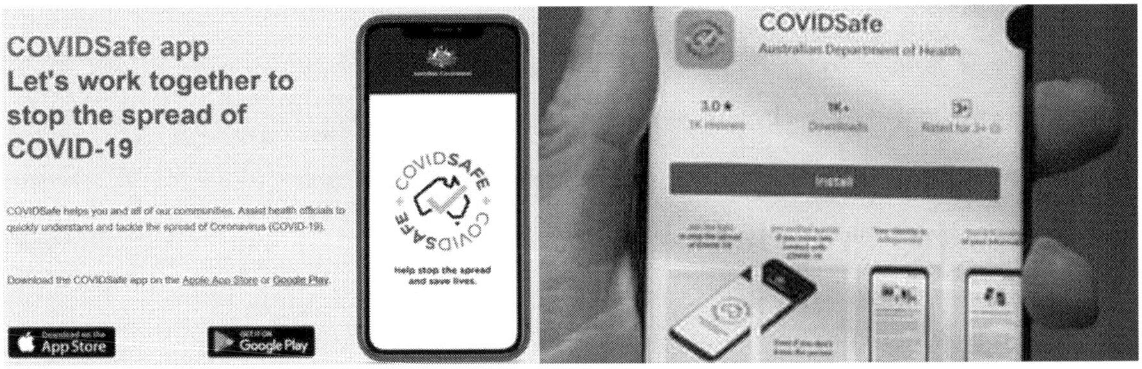

The Australian government is urging people, but not mandatory as many opposed to its intrusion of personal privacy, to install the app into their smartphone to allow the authority to track, detect and give early warnings in order to intervene the potential clustering outbreak from escalating beyond control.

Initiating by a "digital handshake" via the bluetooth and stored contact data from infected patients, user can immediately be notified when he is near to any infected person for more than 15 minutes. The app does not track locality and it seek consent from COVID-19 patients first before sharing their privacy data publicly as governed by their personal privacy data protection regulations.

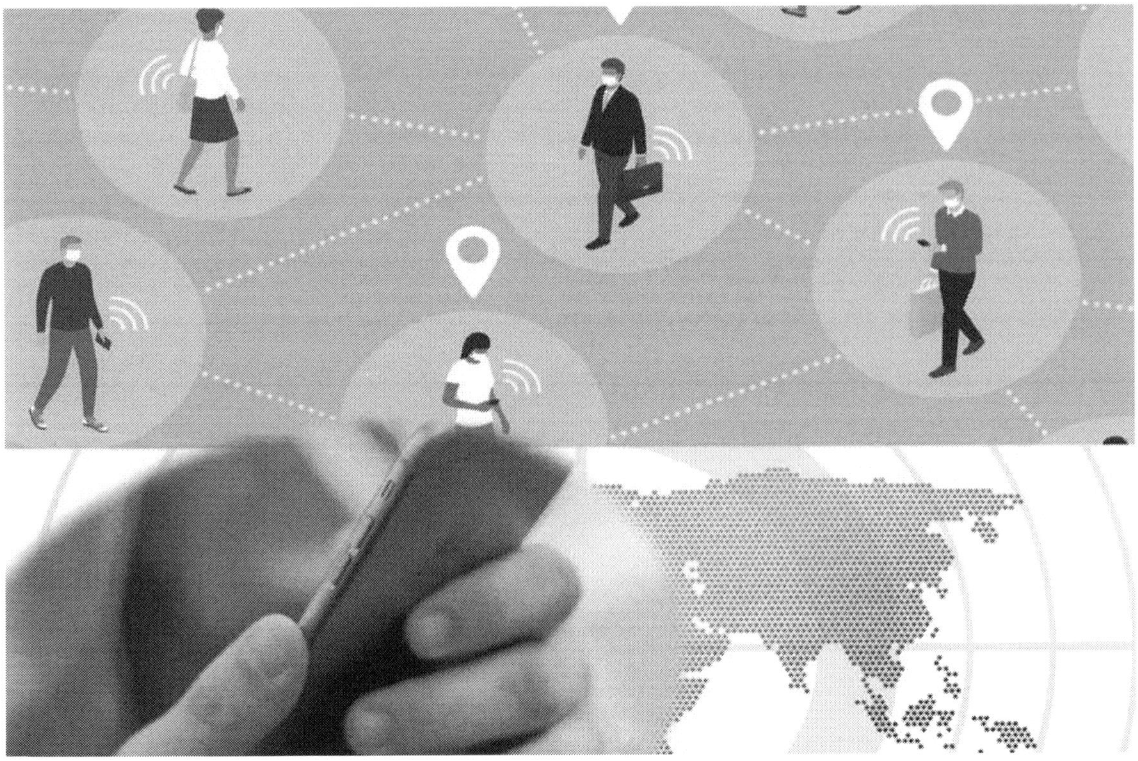

DIY Surgical Face Mask and Face Shield Visor

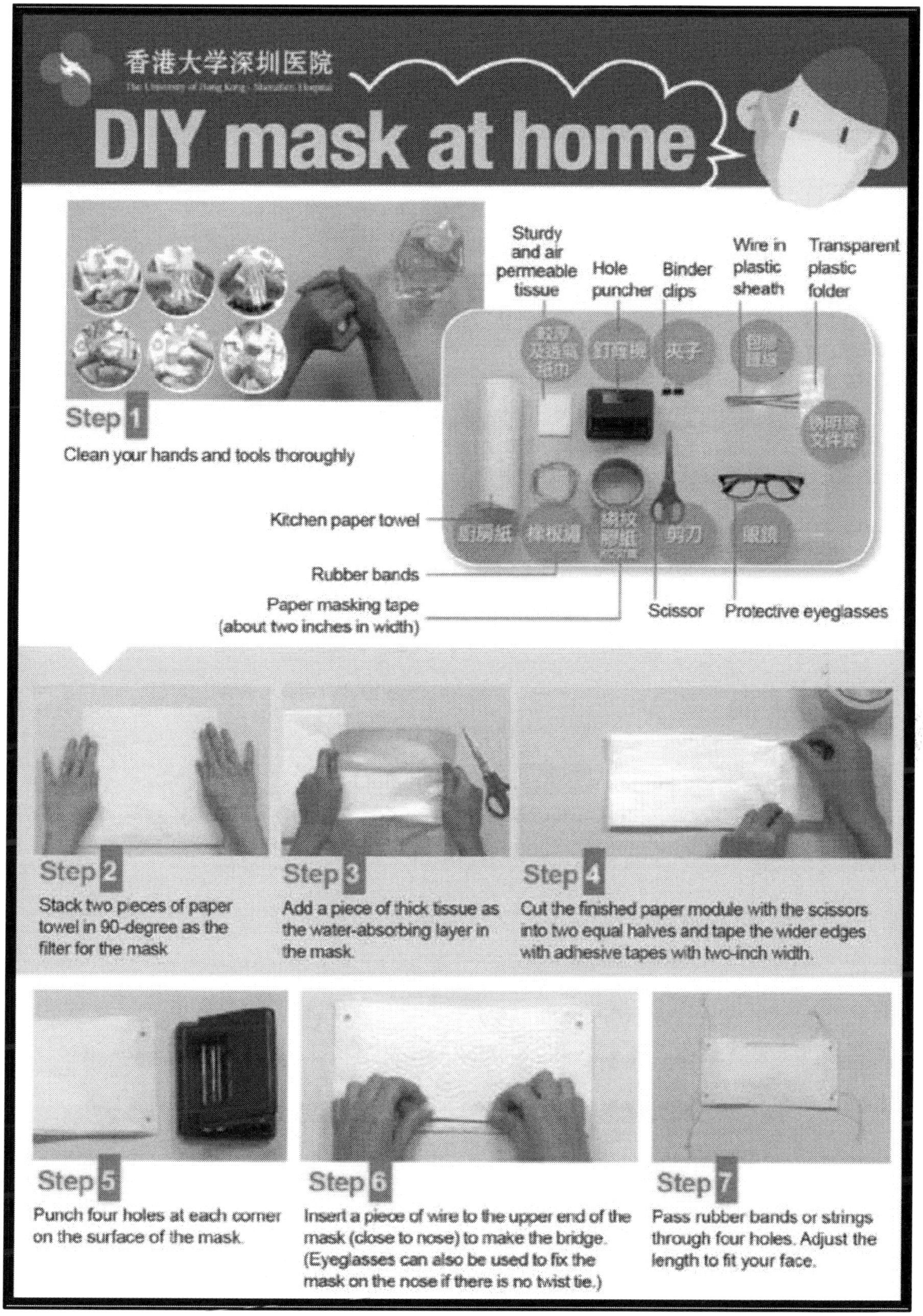

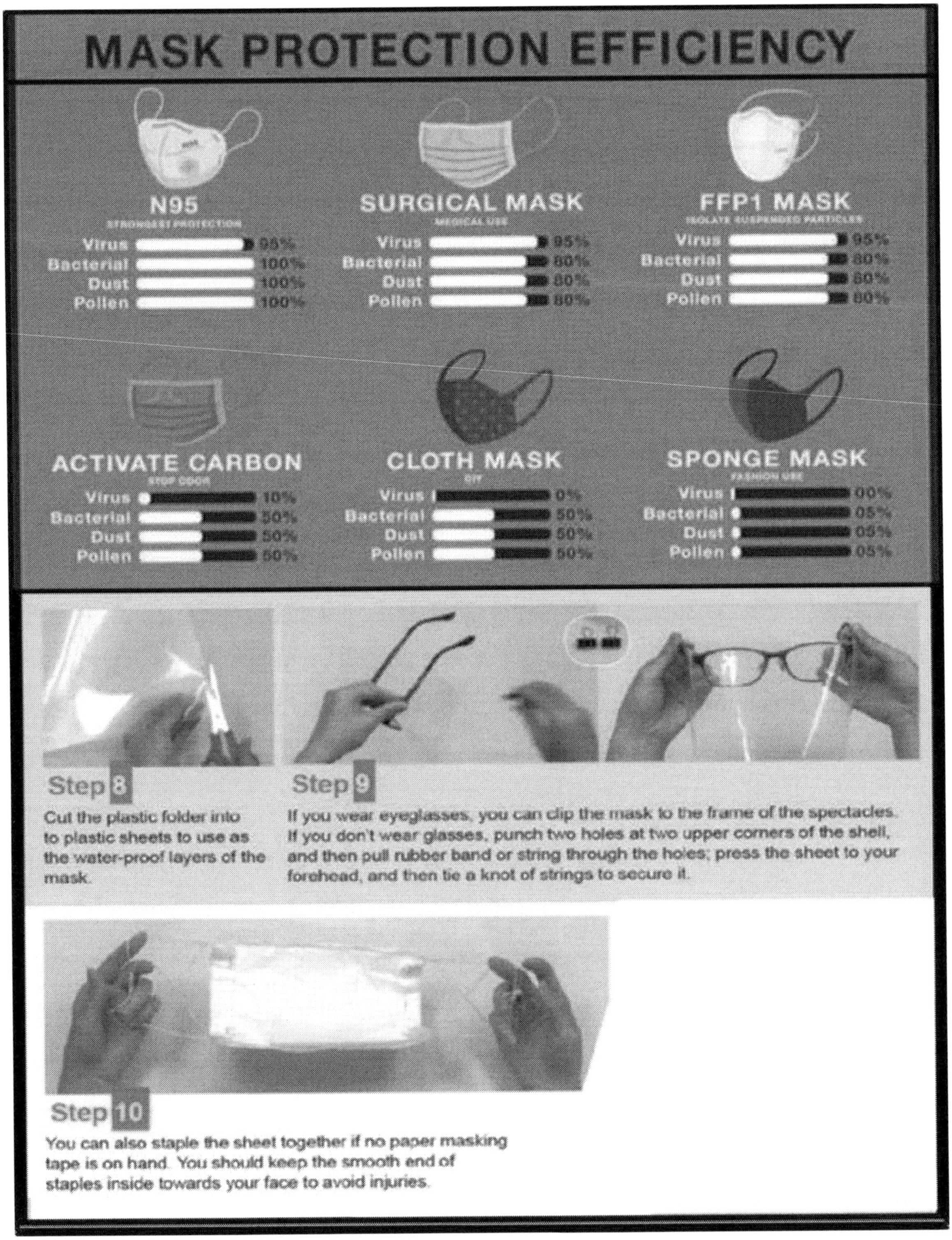

Be responsible and wear a mask when out and about. Dispose used mask in a closed rubbish bin. Do not throw it on the ground such that the cats and dogs can get infected by your irresponsible action!

Microorganism Facts For Kids

G20 Leaders Health Funding Pledge

Facing the common enemy of the novel coronavirus pandemic across the globe, G-20's was set up on 26 March 2020 as a global humanity responsibility to save the world economy from economic recession.

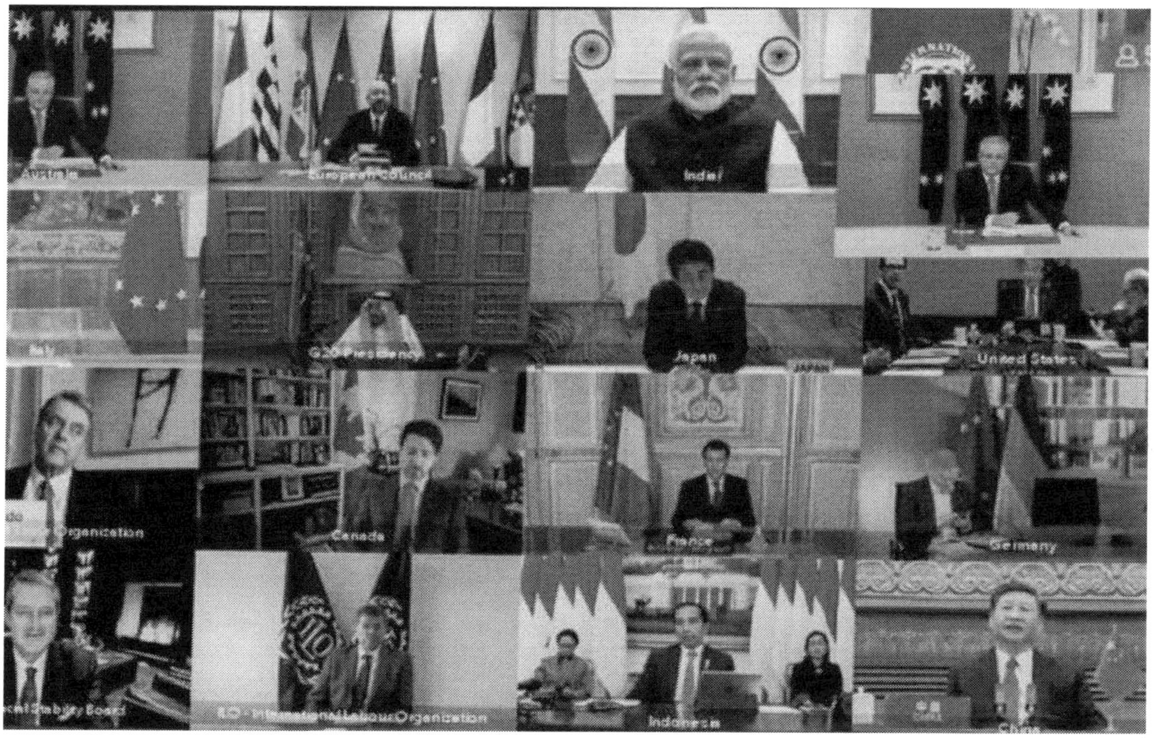

Country leaders all come together as a united frontier in response to the pandemic at a special teleconference summit in a joint statement to save the world from this national pandemic.

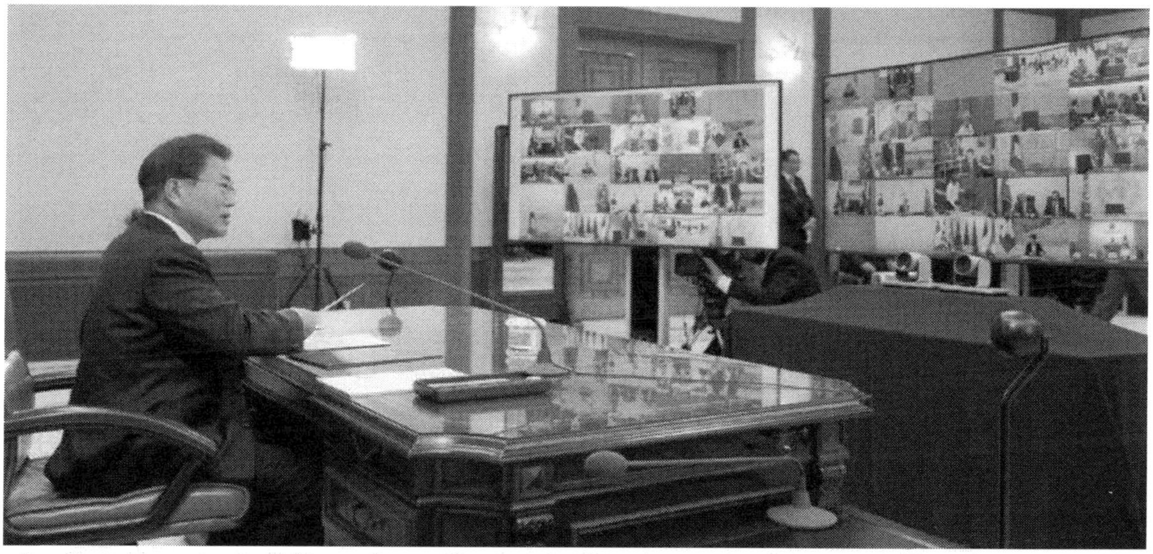

President Moon Jae-in (left) speaking with other G-20 leaders during the special teleconference summit.

The G-20 group leaders have pledged to inject US$5 trillion fiscal stimulus spending aids to help restore the confidence in the global economy in the wake of the pandemic crisis and also seeking support in significant areas like nation healthcare sectors to ensure a continuity flow of vital medical supplies and essential goods and services to pass through borders without any government's interferences and to quickly resolve the disruption of the global supply chain. Besides massive funding, supportive actions are also needed from multilateral coordination efforts in helping globally to save jobs and businesses across borders to maintain continuity of essential trades flow.

Novel coronavirus knows no boundaries. A preparedness robust plan to ensure global food supplies must get ready in action as more countries adopt lockdown policies in spite the fear that supply chain is beginning to feel the impact due to the slowing down in the shipping industry which causes a disruption to the logistical areas that lead to the food shortage supplies across the globe.

WHO leader, Tedros, seeks G-20 group leaders in response to quickly speed up the funding and shipment of PPE for healthcare workers in Africa, Ethiopia, where the communities are poor and lacking healthcare facilities on site, mounting many infection cases and death tolls at an alarming rate to the threat of the coronavirus infections. "A ticking time bomb in Africa," as pointed out by the worried scientist.

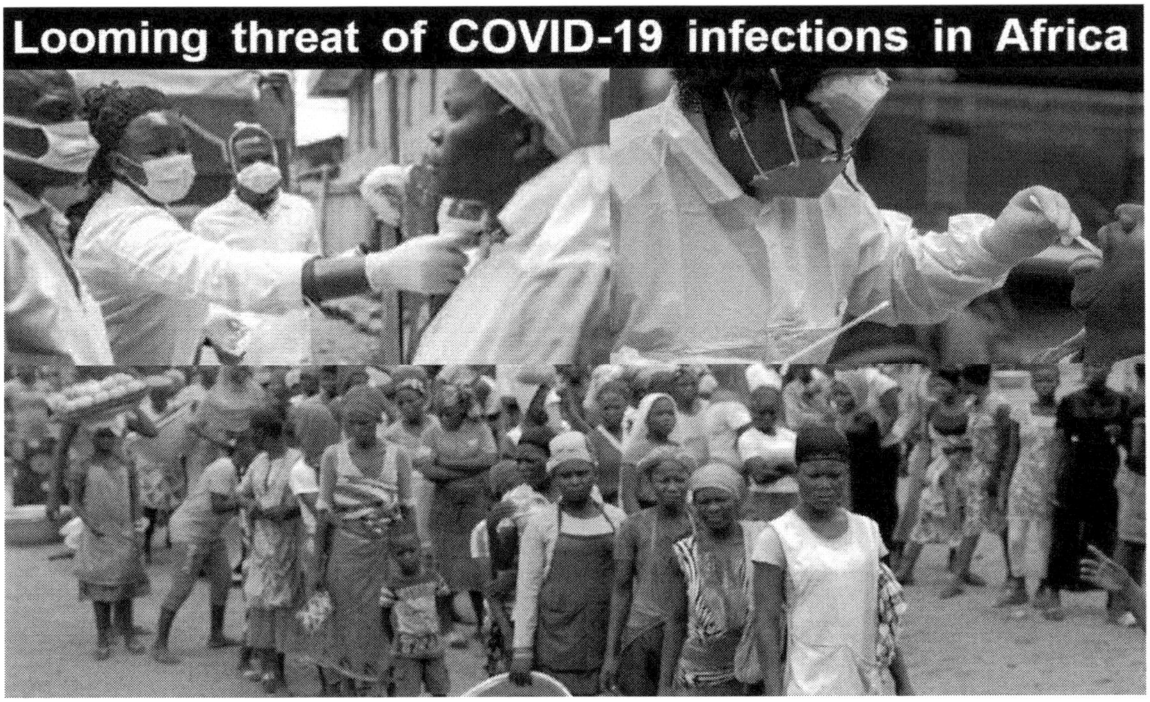

MICROORGANISM FACTS FOR KIDS

Facing the Pandemic

Lockdown Measures

1. Clean and Disinfect Smartphone

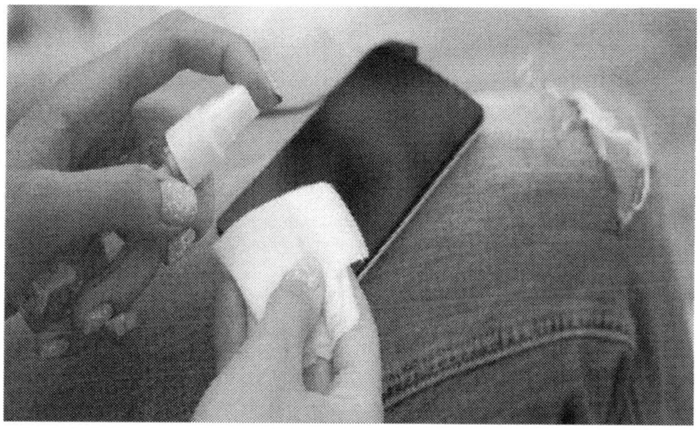

One area that we normally overlook in our personal hygiene is we normally forget to clean our smartphone.

Use a cloth wet with alcohol to wipe and clean it at least once a day as viruses and bacteria can stay up there for 96 hours.

2. Observe Personal Hygiene

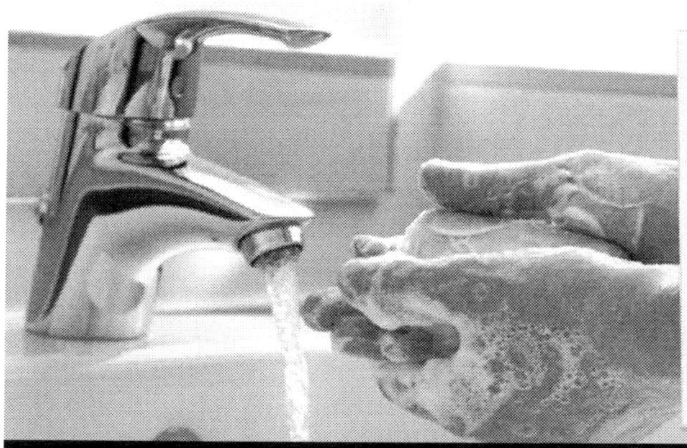

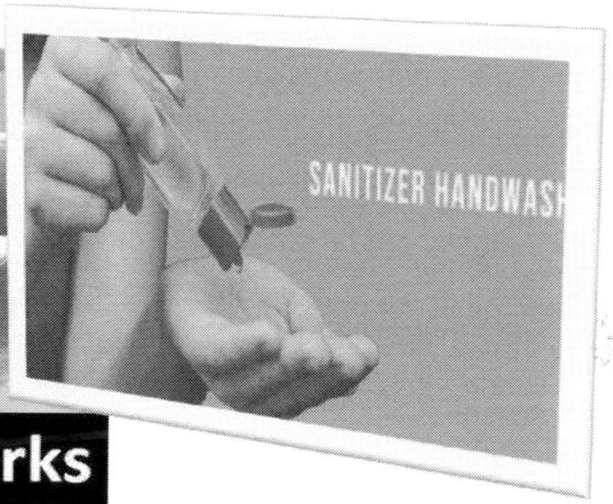

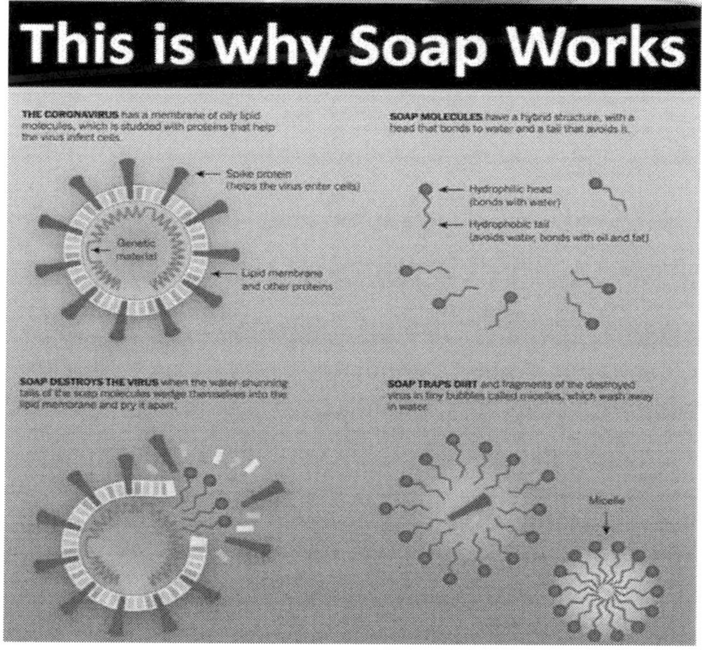

Always wash hand with soap and water frequently to get rid of any germs sticking onto your hands.

If there is no water around, use hand sanitizer instead, but must have at least 70% alcohol contents' based in order to effectively kill the germs.

3. Carry out Self-Check and Monitoring

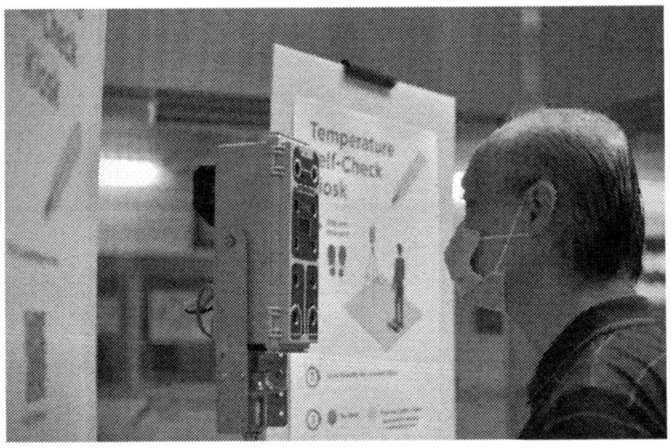

Self-monitoring our own temperature twice daily. Watch out for symptoms like fever, sore throat, eye pain, dry cough, chest pain, breathing difficulties and loss of taste from your tongue or smell. If any of these suspecting symptom occurs, see a doctor to have it checked.

4. Borders Shut to Curb the Virus Spread

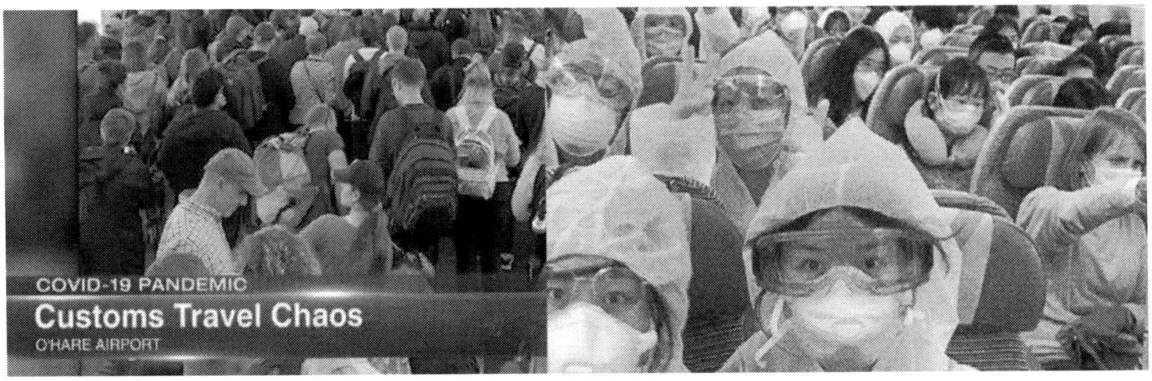

All borders, land and sea, remain closed until further notice. At the beginning of the pandemic, many are seen rushing at the last minute announcement saw airport chaos with people dashing and dragging along their luggage to catch one of the few planes flying back home.

Everybody feared of not able to get a flight back home. Flying in the midst of a worldwide pandemic is costly, demanding and dangerously risky under cramping and enclosed cabins for a long journey back home.

All permit pass holders were barred from entering or transiting over.

5. Work from Home, Home-Based-Learning

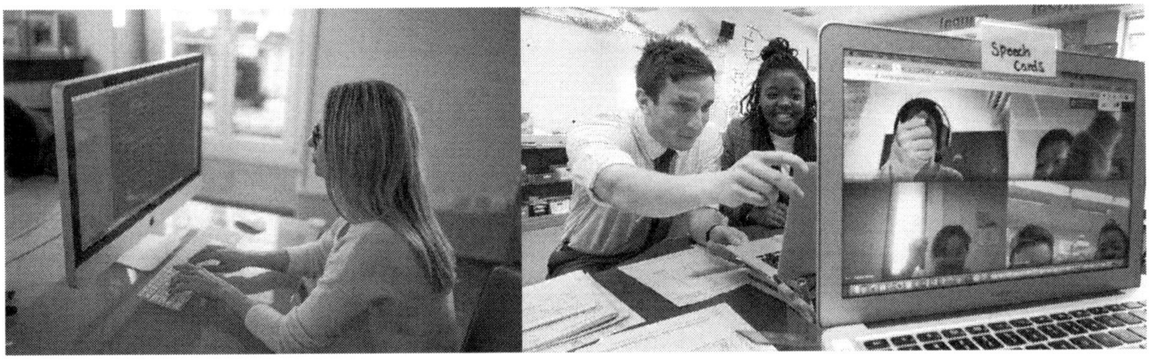

Telecommuting were strongly encouraging working people and educationist to use internet broadband technology to replace their old way of working style at work and in school learning process.

6. Avoid Physical Contact

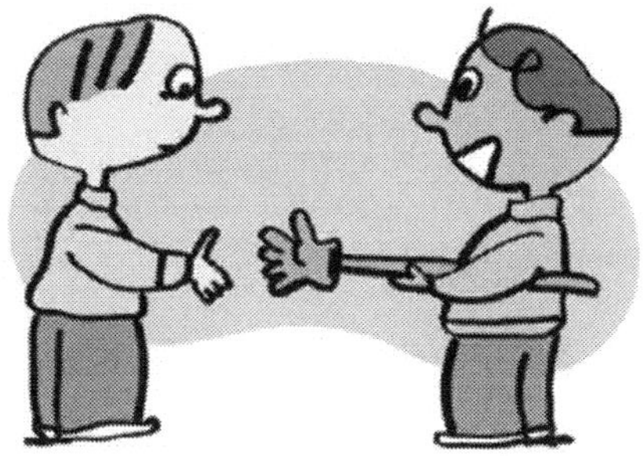

No large group or religious gatherings, standing in pairs or mingling with social community, but instead head straight home after carrying out essential services.

7. Stay Home Orders

Except doing essential work and buying food, there is no dining out but only takeaway meals are allowed. When out, mask wearing is compulsory. Violators will be fined and those foreign workers found breaching their stay-home notices will have their work permit pass cancelled and permanently barred from coming in to work.

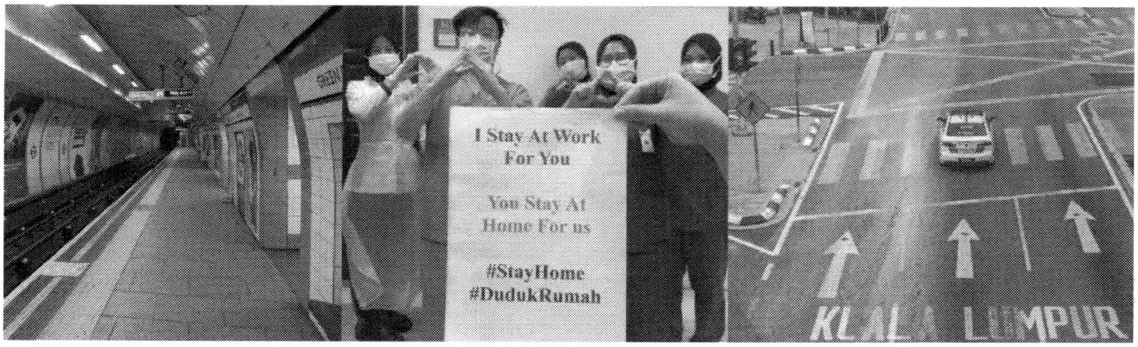
I Stay At Work
For You
You Stay At
Home For us
#StayHome
#DudukRumah

8. Social Distancing Responsibility

Social distancing measures kicked in to limit crowds at essential service places like supermarket stores, F&B outlets, public transport etc.

All entertainment venues, museums and attractions places and tuition centres are to remain closed until further notice.

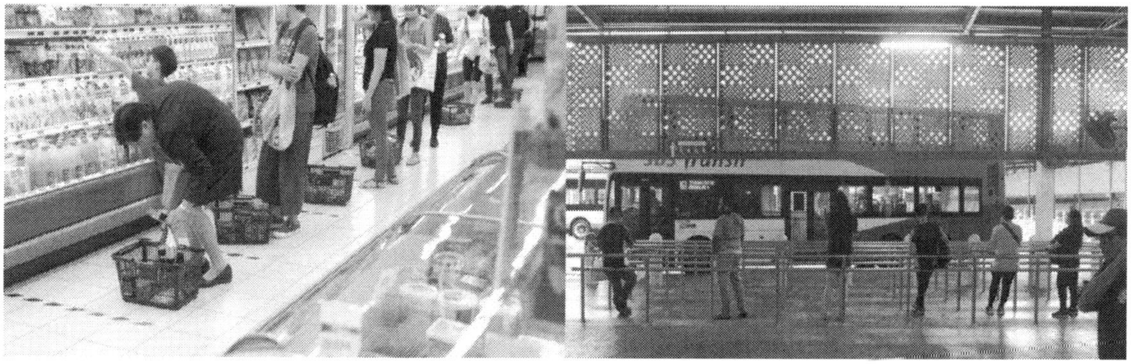

9. Taking Care of the Elders and the Weak

Social community care groups and additional helpline services are setting up to assist them. They can always call and ask for assistance if they are alone and need help to see to their personal needs, daily meals and doctor appointments

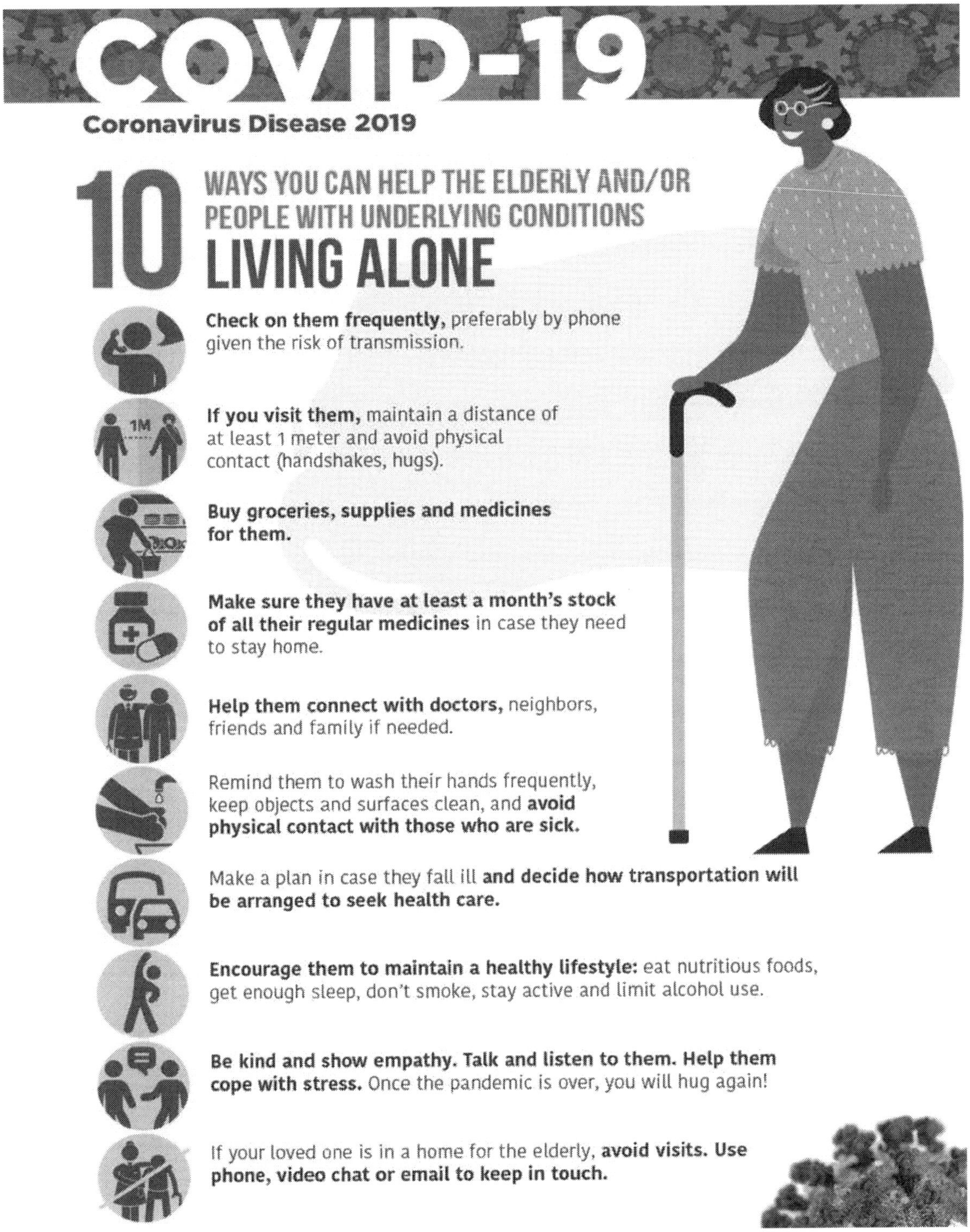

10. Self-Quarantine Advice

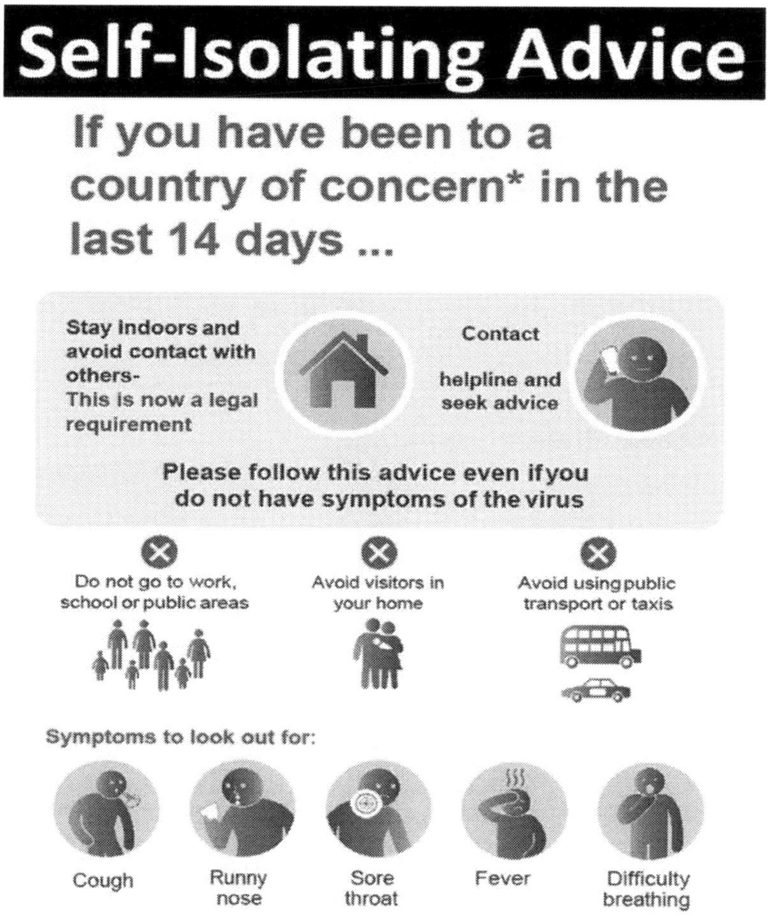

When coming back from oversea, one must impose own self-isolation for minimum of 14 days:

- Coming back from oversea trip
- Living with an infected patient
- Coming near or in close proximity with COVID patient.

Self-Isolation Rules for living

1. Single and living alone

- Don't let anyone like friends, colleagues and family to visit you
- Strictly confine and stay at home all the times for 14 days
- Strictly no friends, colleagues and family gatherings around you

2. Sharing with roommates or living with partner or family

- Self-isolate yourself for a minimum of 14 days if you have contracted mild symptoms.
- Confine yourself to a room alone. No sharing the room with others, not even your partner.
- Always wear mask to cover your mouth when coughing and sneezing.
    - Wash hands thoroughly with soap and water frequently.
    - Wear disposable gloves when getting a glass of water.
    - Wipe touched surfaces.

Microorganism Facts For Kids

The Fighting Spirit

So take care of yourself first.

Protect the elderly, and stay home!

Stay safe, stay healthy, stay positive and stay survive.

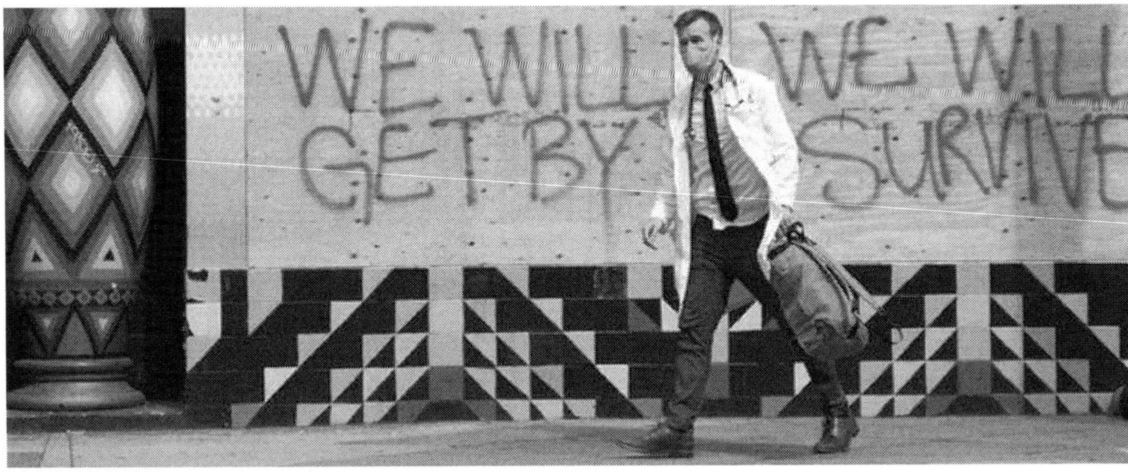

Because as we know it, the world needs you, and you needs the world as much as we do!

Together, we can conquer this coronavirus pandemic!

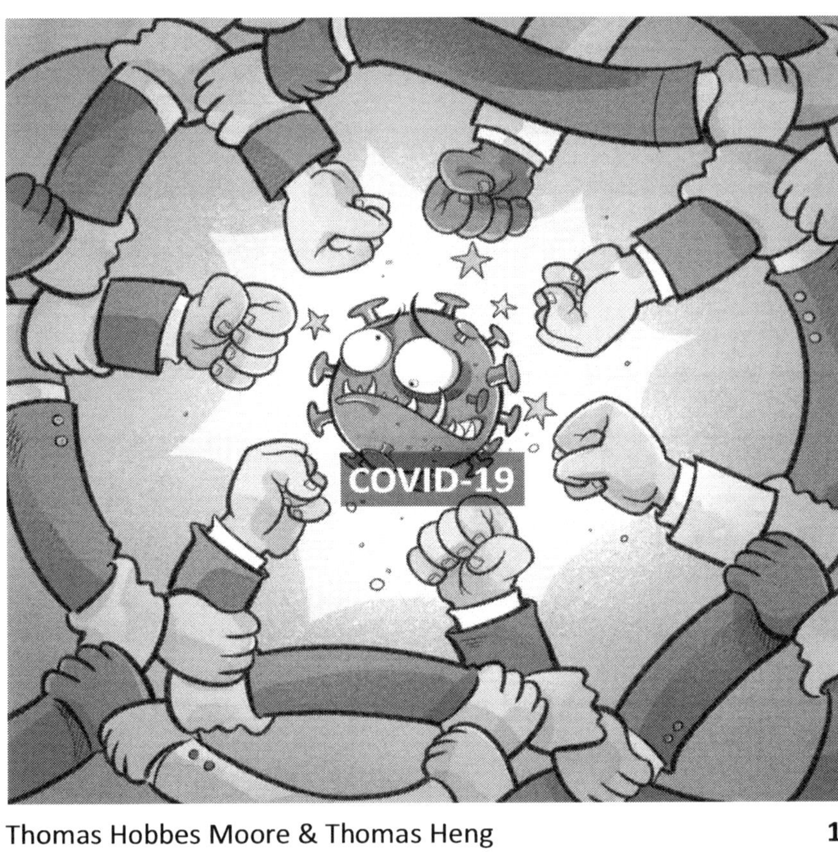

Microorganism Facts For Kids

The Untold Sacrifices & Unsung Heroes

There were many untold sacrifices from the frontline healthcare workers as they soldiered on the fight with COVID-19 day in and day out. Within the sprawling hospital compound, many were hard at work, quietly working behind the scenes donning on the goggles, shower cap, gloves, N95 mask and plastic gown to protect themselves where each and every individual played a different role as the infectious cases increased daily.

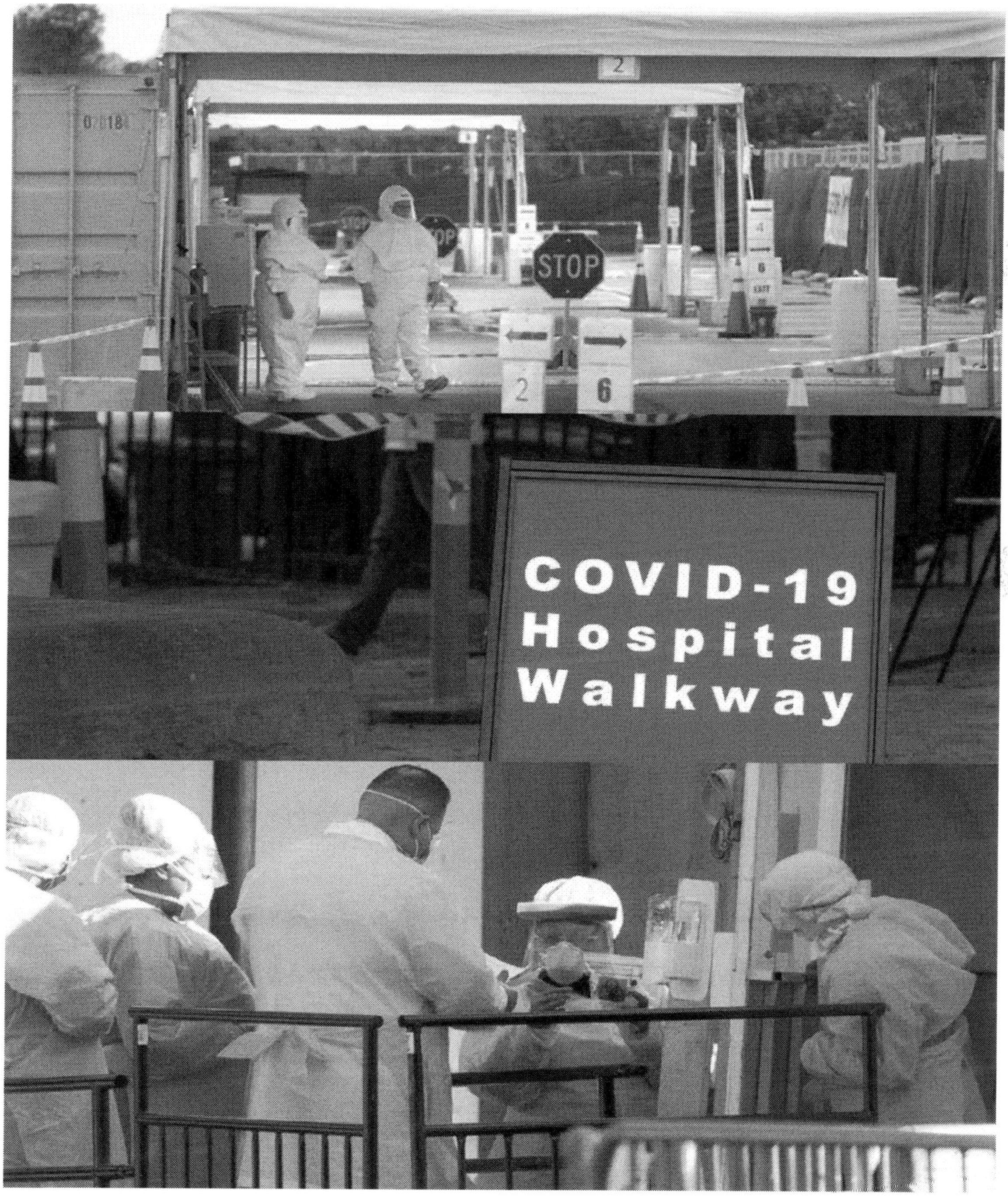

Microorganism Facts For Kids

As the outbreak escalated, there were many sick patients coming forward to the hospital seeking for treatment. Barricades and signages were putting up, directing everyone entering the main entrance must have their temperature taken and screened. Workload and duties of the healthcare workers were drastically increased.

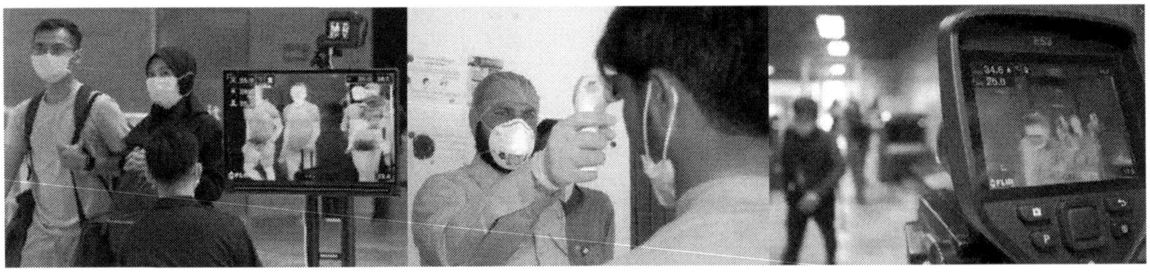

Some transport swabbed samples, cleaned the wards, escorted the patients, and changed the laundry. Essential services like porters, housekeepers, security officers, linen services etc. were the ones that we normally took their services for granted and did not pay any attention to it.

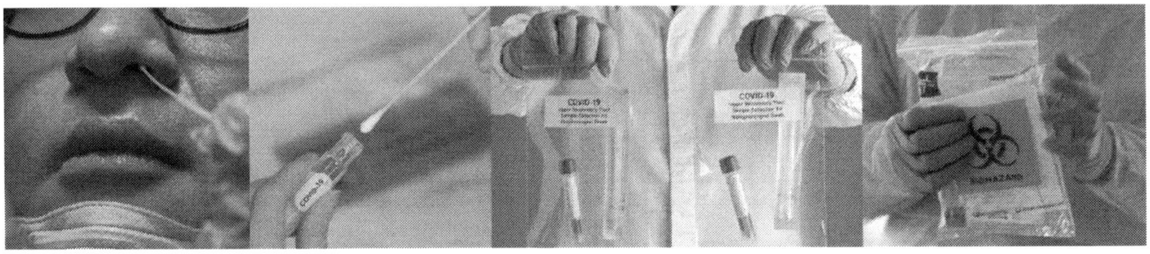

For instance the housekeeper, the one that played the role of making the place safe and ensuring that the rooms, the toilet, the ward area, the corridor area, countertops as well as the staff pantry were cleaned and disinfected all the surfaces to keep them germs free.

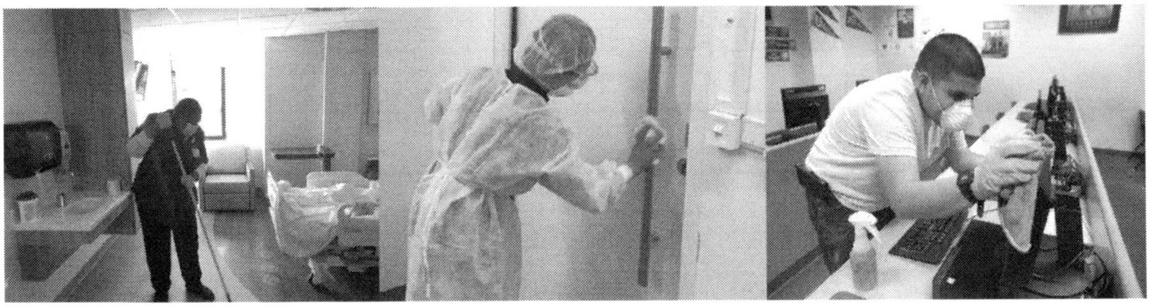

When the patients were discharged, they would come in to carry out a thorough cleaning so that the ward was ready for the next patient admission. Even when there was an extreme discharges of patient, they would still manage to overcome the extra workload as they fully understood their role and function without any complaints.

Many even went to the extent of cutting short their lunch break when there were times many patients discharged from the wards on the same day.

Many expressed concerned and said the same notion, “Nothing to worry about, we have to do our duties. We are happy to help the sick patients. Our role is to make and keep the place safe and clean for everybody and everywhere. When the place is cleaned and tidied, we are happy.”

Some even came with more touching expressions, “Everyone works in the hospital is a frontliner. We are frontliners and we do our part in helping one another as part of the team too. Bedsheets, blankets, towels, pyjamas for patients, curtains, and linens in the wards are all under our care.”

During this crisis, we could see many healthcare workers doing their jobs in a responsible and serious attitudes in attending to their sick patients' needs. Across the globe, people were thankful to their healthcare workers on the COVID-19 frontline and tons of thankful notes with gifts of appreciation from the public were posted and had given them a positive perspectives and motivation actions to keep their morale high and to continue working together as a unified team spirit to overcome their job stress and tiredness in fighting the bug.

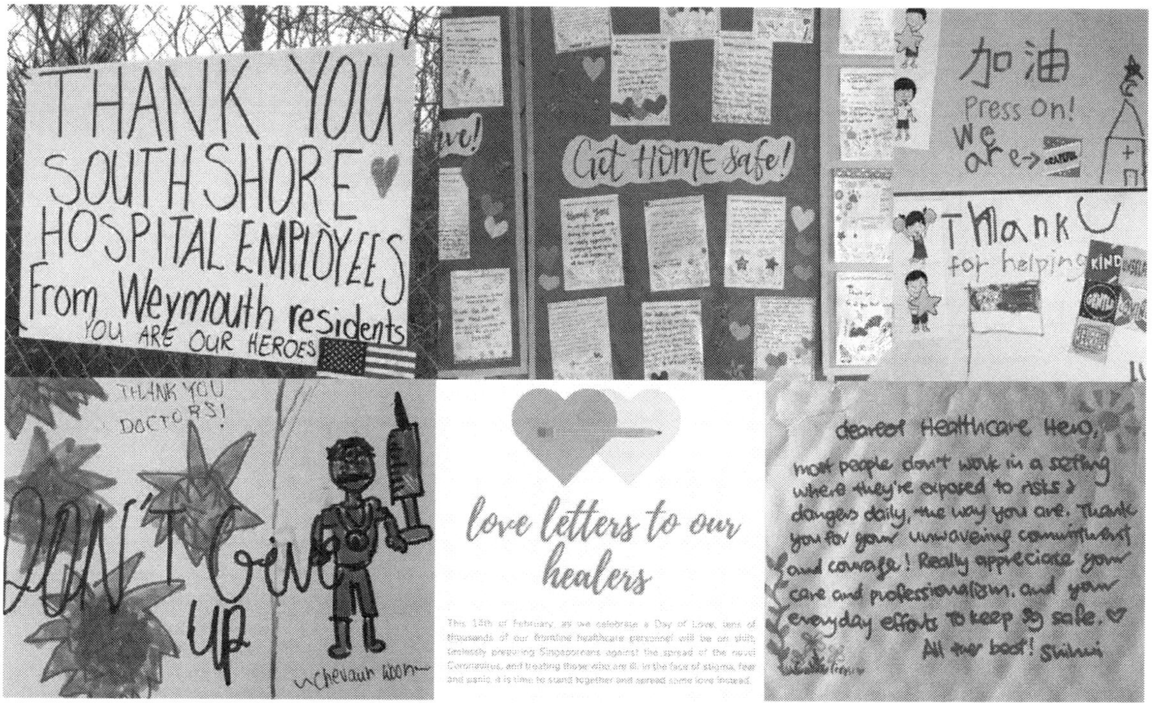

Some kind souls from the public had offered to send in free food daily on a voluntarily basis in a way of recognising their immense sacrifices, invaluable dedication and hardwork they had put in.

MICROORGANISM FACTS FOR KIDS

Everything in the hospital's protocols had changed eversince the pandemic hit the shores and everybody was facing the same challenges.

For instance:

1. To prevent germs cross-contamination when handling dirty linen that might come from the infected patients, the team member wore T-Shirt and medical scrub pants rather than the standard uniforms that were previously issued by the hospital.

   While wheeling the COVID-19 patients before and after the screening centre, they were required to put on a full PPE attires. In a day, they probably had to change many times on the PPE attires while patients were being transported within the hospital.

2. Before transferring a COVID-19 patient out of the ward, the porter had to communicate with the officer at the infectious control centre and the different departments for clearance and the transfer routes to be taken.

   Blockages and signages had to put up along the transfer routes to inform people that the COVID-19 patient's transfer was in process.

3. The supervising officers-in-charge for instance the security and updating officers were required to devise a proper planning schedules and duties' roosters to internal and external outsourced officers to know exactly what duties they were to perform in the day ahead within the hospital complex.

In the beginning, new comers were finding it troublesome and uncomfortable to change the PPE attires many times in a day. But as time passed by, they began to understand the need of keeping themselves safe from the virus at the end of the day for himself, his family and others.

Community isolation facilities were being set up elsewhere to make up the shortfall of hospital beds so that ambulances can make the necessary transfers in process.

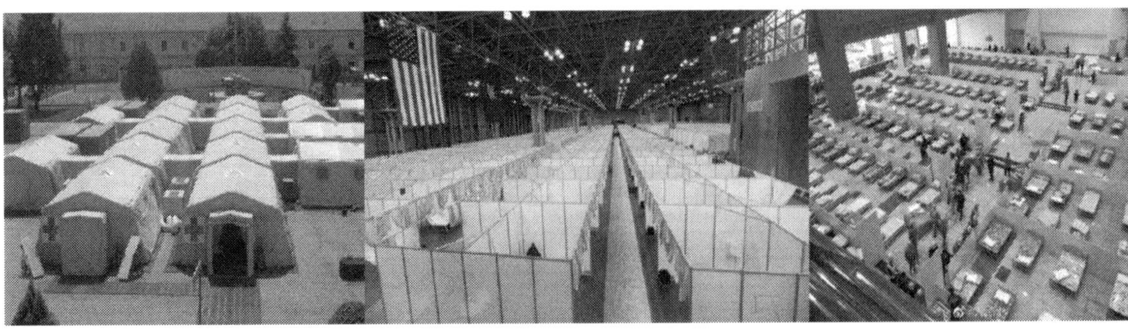

Medical workers Bitter Realities

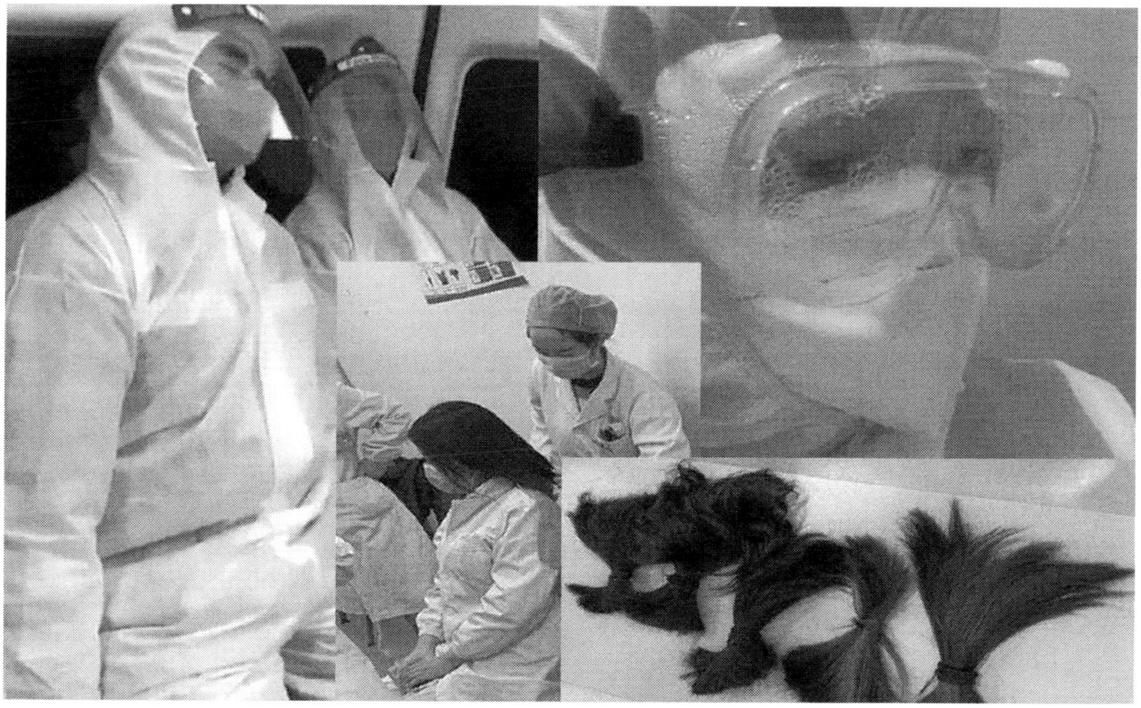

All the medical frontliners are truly amazing and deserving our recognition and respect for their dedication and sacrifices they have to make and placing their own health risk on the frontline of coronavirus to save the sick patients. Each and every single of them went above the call of duty, especially the ladies' nurses and doctors with long hairs all have their full head of hairs shaved off completely and become bald in order to reduce the risk of cross-contamination from the virus. They put on adult diapers and some even take birth control pills to delay their menstrual cycle and counting. After layering themselves on their protective gear, they enter the wards with full dedication of their duty and optimism to fight the coronavirus battle. They are our true heroes and GREAT warriors for humanity indeed!

Once inside the wards, doctors and nurses alike do not have the time to

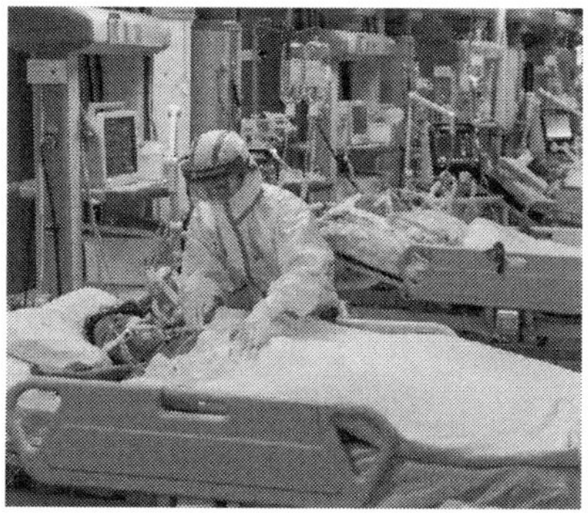

go to the bathroom to relieve themselves, to eat or drink. They have to withstand an unpleasant and prolonged working hours in wearing the same protective suits while making their rounds to check, monitor and even trying to save infected patients from terrible breathing difficulties and massive heart attack occurrences.

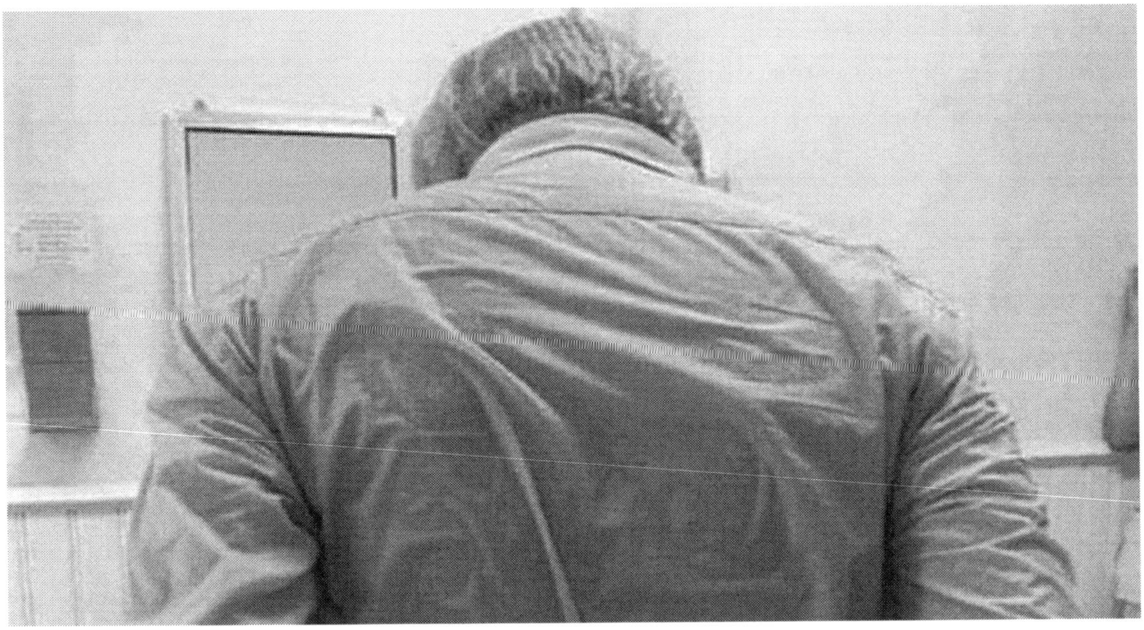

The doctor is completely exhausted after working long hour of gruelling shift and not able to breathe freely. Not only that, they have to withstand skin irritations from their protective goggles and masks, and also their body itchiness from their protective suits which are extremely hot, suffocating and uncomfortable to wear. Signs of skin irritation and bloody marks from their masks are clearly shown on their faces and noses' bridges due to long hours of usage.

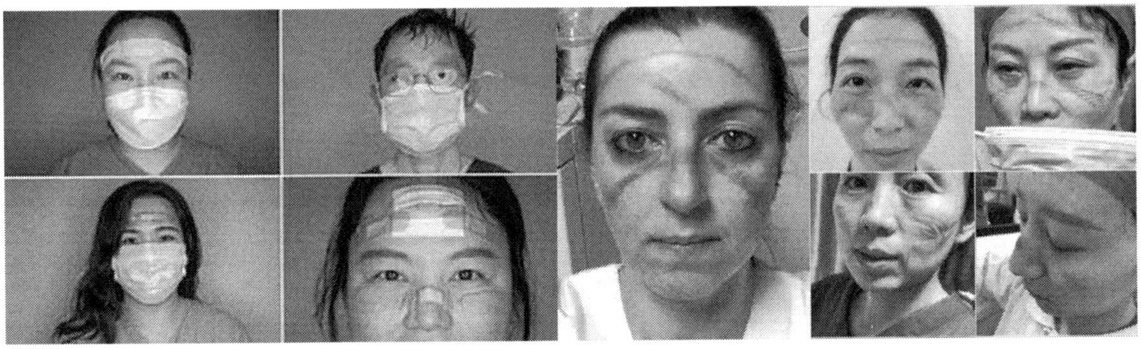

All the medical workers are working round-the-clock in the wake of the coronavirus crisis at the hospitals that many of them after the shift are staying back behind, finding a little corner area to rest or sleep until the next shift and then repeats the whole cycle again. This is the bitter reality of the hardship that are facing by the medical workers while protecting and caring for the infected sick patients, a call beyond duty and dedication.

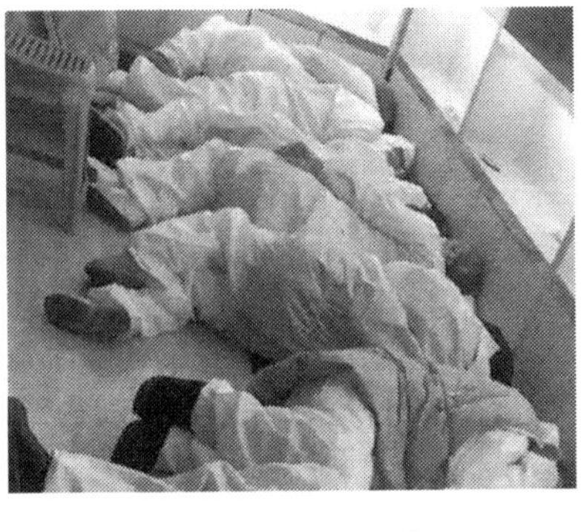

The Whistleblower

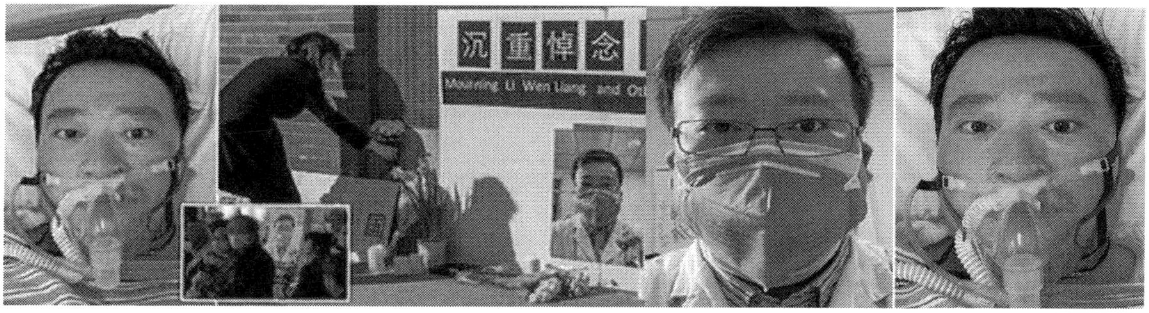
沉重悼念

Li Wen Liang, a 34 years old ophthalmologist doctor married with 2 children is a coronavirus whistleblower in the early stage of coronavirus. He sounded an early warning to the Wuhan community in December 2019 about a possible outbreak of an illness that had similarly resemblance's behaviour of SARS-CoV-1 outbreak in 2003 epidemic. His warnings was rubbished by the local police as rumour-mongering and was given a stern warning with meting out serious punishment if his action repeated again.

A glaucoma patient happened to be treated by him on 10 January 2020 at his hospital got him infected. His diagnosis and test results later came out confirming positive to coronavirus on January 30. Outrage and grief of his death angered the public over the government tight reins of information that caused an igniting spark to the Chinese to demand for freedom of speech. After his death, Li Wen Liang was looked upon as an unsung hero of China by the Chinese who had made sacrifices and one who is willing to speak out the truth. On February 7, he died from the coronavirus infection at the hospital. News of his death was made known through the Press and picked up by the netizens that later on became the top read topics on Weibo dashboard with over 1 billion online viewers. Many went to his funeral site to light up a candle and pay tribute to the hero, some exclaiming "You are the beam of light in the night!" while others posted poems, photos and drawings saluting him for his courageous act of speaking out the truth.

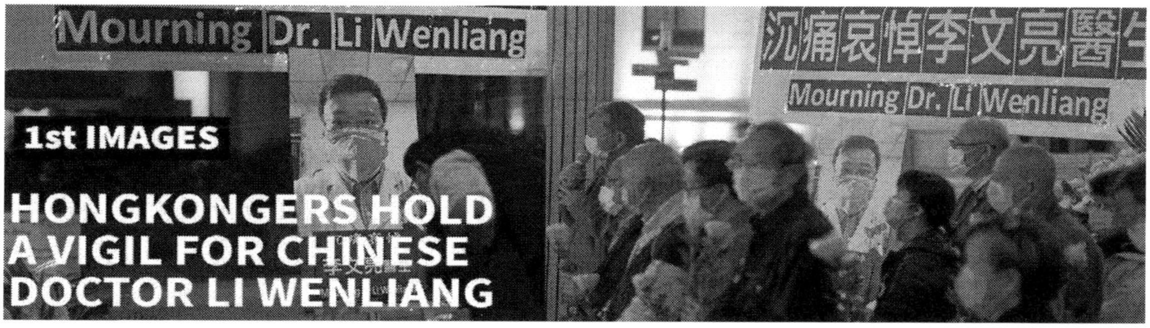
Mourning Dr. Li Wenliang
沉痛哀悼李文亮醫
Mourning Dr. Li Wenliang
1st IMAGES
HONGKONGERS HOLD
A VIGIL FOR CHINESE
DOCTOR LI WENLIANG

Reshaping of Consumer and Business Behaviour

More Localised Production

The lesson that we had learned from the pandemic had clearly highlighted to us the heavy risks of having to rely on distant foreign producers of critical mass production on the importance of certain basic needs of medical PPE, medicine, microchips and food supplies in the sudden reoccurrence of such pandemic outbreaks in the near future.

National governments have to adopt a need to diversify the network chain of regional suppliers in terms of time deliverance and the requirement of domestic production on critical goods and the new impetus for the local private entities sectors to diversity supply lines as well. Companies may need to reconsider and foreseeing the future stockpiling of greater quantity of inventories including critical components in the pipelines.

More Flexible Commuting Options

The economic and social interactions of doing business globally and locally now involve in virtual internet meetings and working from home. Both employees and employers have truly learned to adopt the possibility of working from home or some other off-site premises rather than going back to the old ways of staying in the office working till late nights.

As long as people are equipped with a laptop or tablet and have a reliable internet connections, business meetings and proposals can still continue to function in today technology. Ultimately, this pandemic crisis has put the world towards a new different pattern of work-life balance.

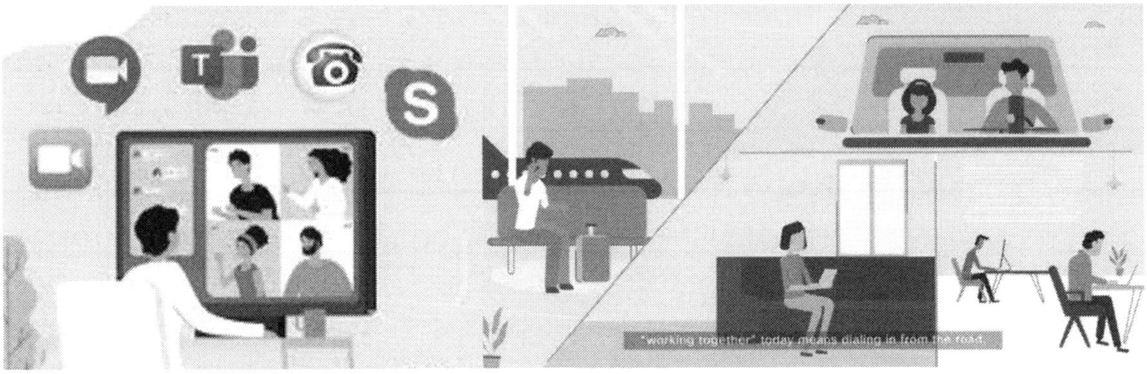

Fewer people need to drive or take public transport to work, and these have turned into a blessing in disguise which make a greater improvement effort to our global warming consequences with less pollution. The sky now seems to look brilliant and bright and not so cloudiness nowadays.

Less Business Travel

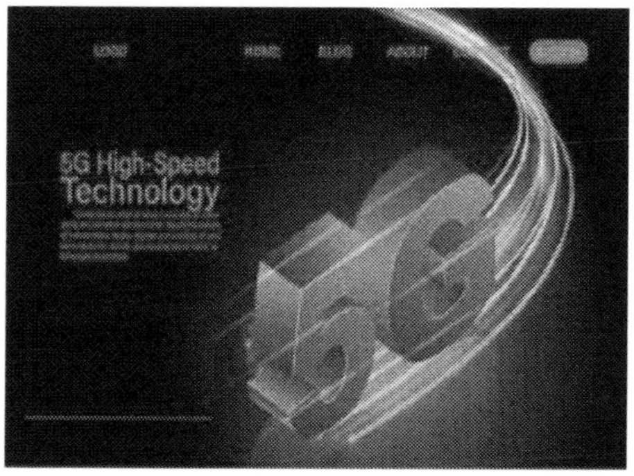

With the world advanced internet technologies with 5G on the pipelines, fewer corporate business travelling by flight may not be necessary as more can adopt virtual internet meetings and webinars via Zoom, Google meetings or Microsoft meetings without the need to travel oversea for business meetings and seminars.

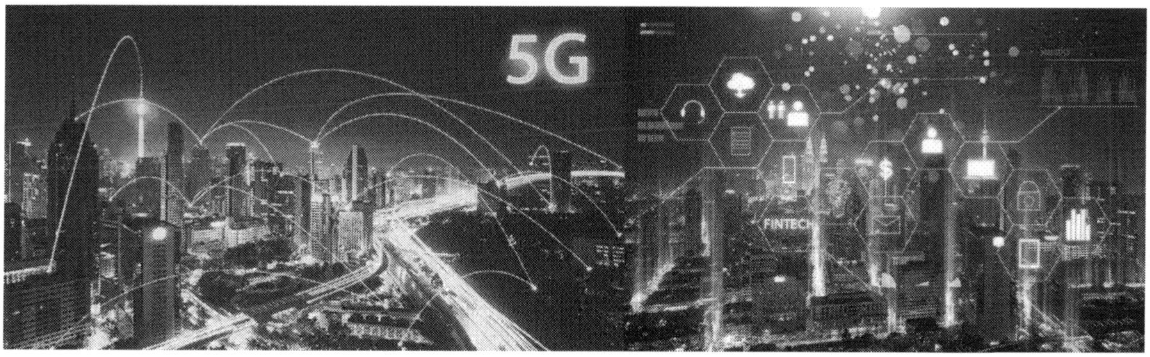

Either for face-to-face meetings or engaging with people as a group, communications via virtual internet meetings can still achieve the same results ultimately.

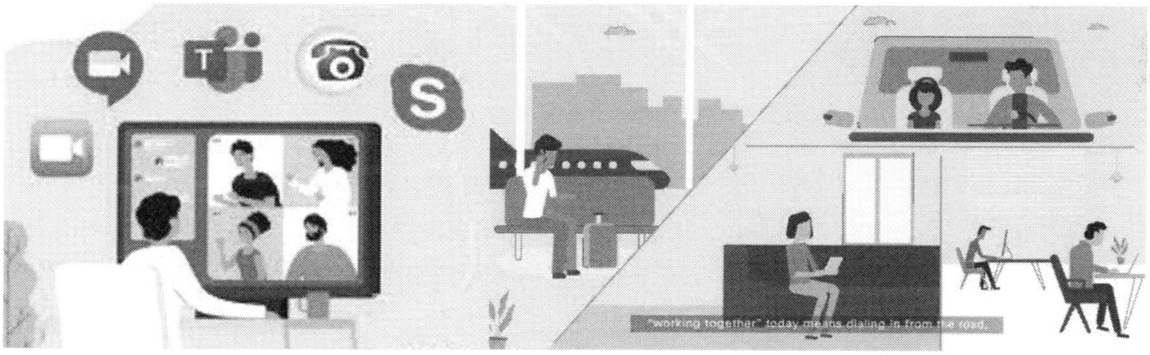

On the contrary, business travel is time consuming and also causing another large expenses to be incurred.

Needless to say, airlines and hotels will be badly affected and come at less in demand. The business structure for most businesses to sustain in today crises will have to re-model and re-design their strategies and manpower relocation.

Retrenchment of employees will see in the last resort of no-solution calls in order to sustain business on-going.

Online Retail Prevails

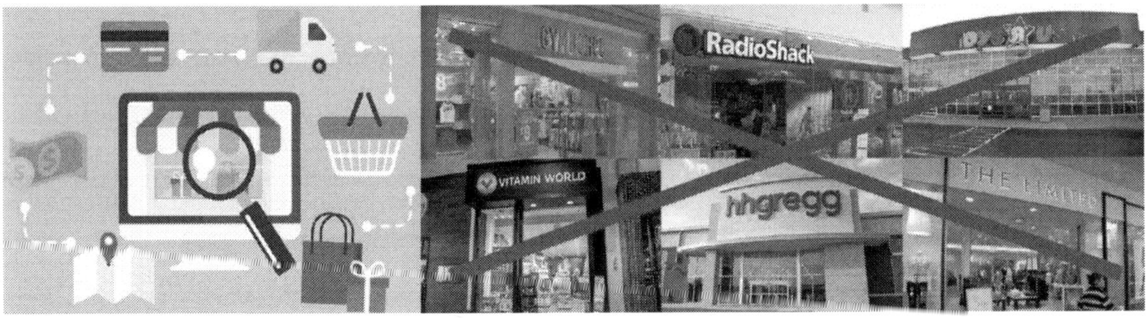

In the past, consumers do their shopping on physical stores. Eversince the emerged pandemic crises, more are turning towards ecommerce online portal instead to do their shopping and opting for online deliveries. As such, online orderings have now become a necessity in today lives and the only option to purchase as more brick-and-mortar stores are now under tremendous pressure and being forced to shut down due to fewer shoppers and are infeasible to sustain businesses with high rentals and struggling to pay off their staff salaries.

Landlord in shopping malls and offices are now finding more difficult to look for tenant replacement for their store fronts this time around. Moreover, the nature of retail has now changed the consumers' mindset from traditional way of buying to online purchase conveniences at a click of a button. As such, there are big implications for tenants who are willing to pay rent on shopping malls concept.

Cash Is King

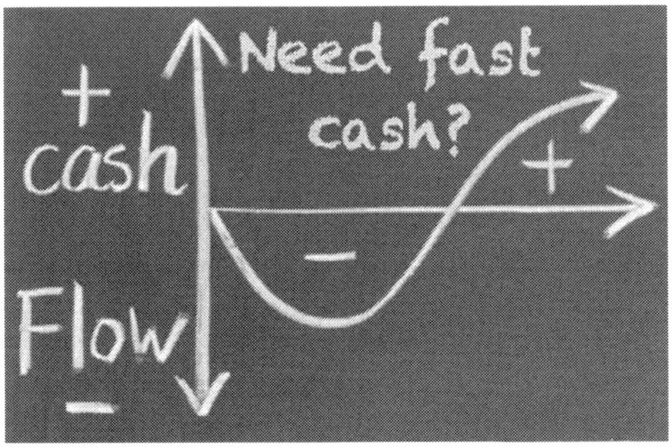

Banks have drastically reduced their loan interest. Not because of seeking out more loaners, but instead they are more worried that many are not able to pay off their loans during this crisis as many businesses shut down have caused job loss and not able to get a job with the kind of salary that the employee is enjoying previously. Getting loan approval from banks is now even harder as bank relation officers will need to thoroughly check through the applicant affordability background. Even so, if the applicant has no problem, the bank will also not grant him the full loan at the most 60% loan amount payable.

As public debt soars to the sky, the private sector might have to de-leverage. For instance, rather than giving out profits as dividends in stock shares, they are now withholding a greater share of corporate earnings instead.

Business Will Never Be the Same As Before

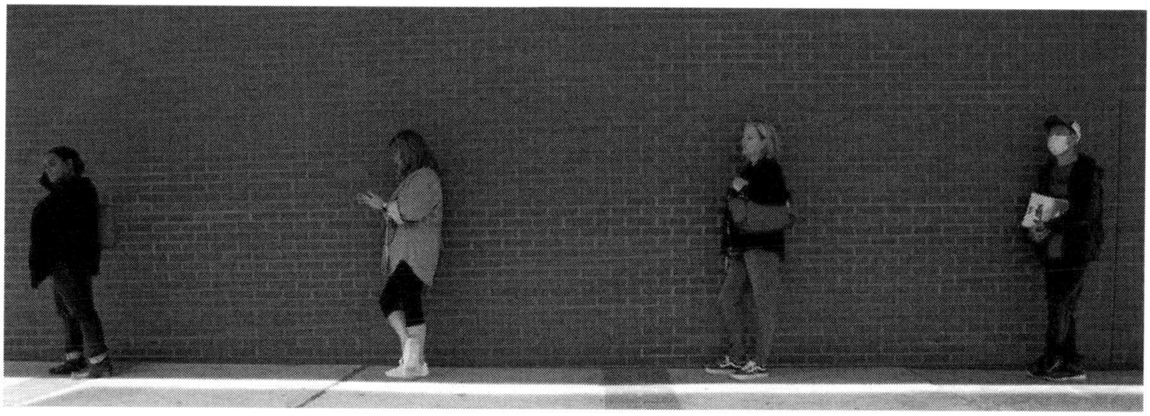

It will not be business as usual after the pandemic crisis. This crisis has now become the biggest hurdle of economic shock since WWII as governments across the globe implement mandatory orders to social isolation measures, shutting down businesses and instructing people to work from home to slow the infection spread of the virus diseases transmitting from human to human.

This so called "isolation economy" has inevitably created a new business model activity boom to food delivery services like Grab, Deliveroo, Amazon Web Services, Zoom Video Communications and Internet Broadband Service Providers to have benefitted significantly to the extent that their delivery schedules may be stressed as many are trying to find a slot for home delivery through online ordering.

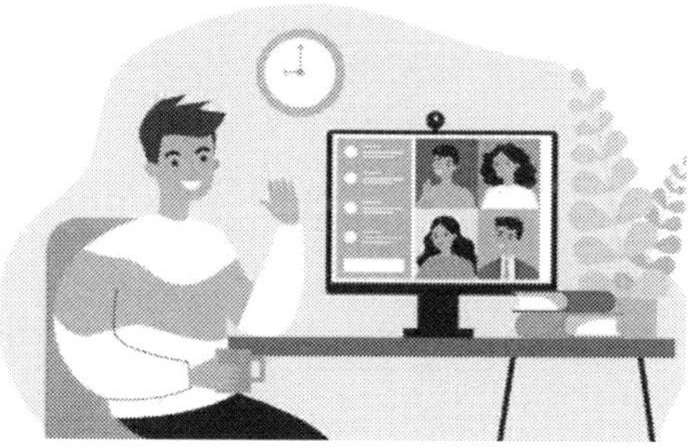

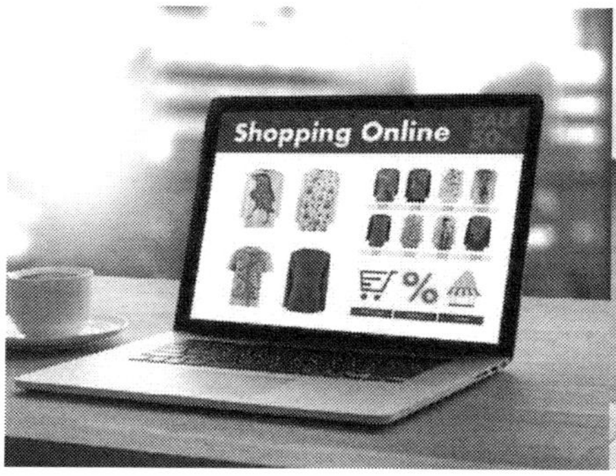

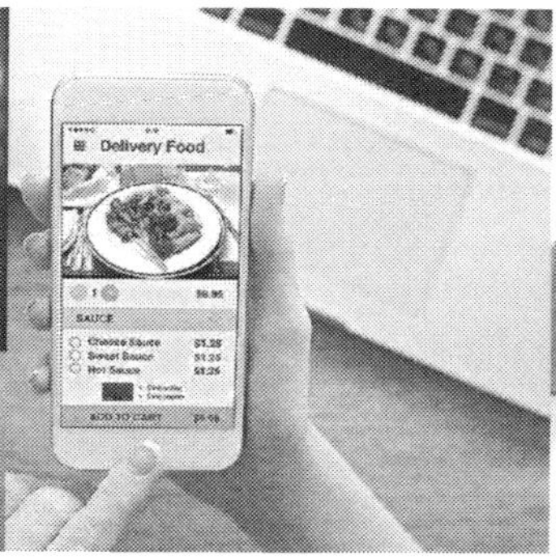

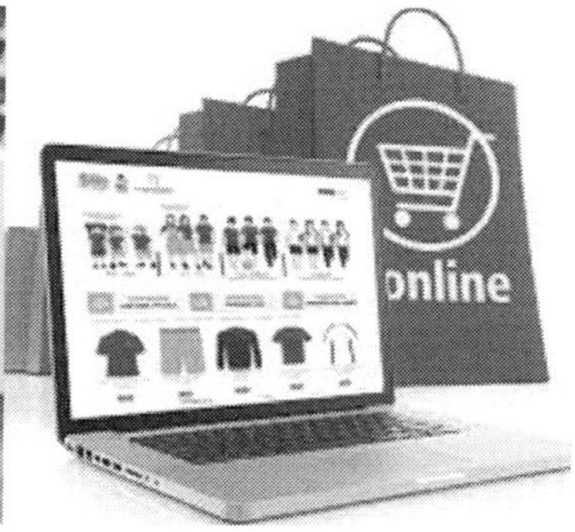

Printed in Great Britain
by Amazon

61364072R00080